How to keep a morning lark quiet a bit longer....

A morning lark is not a child who wakes at 4 A.M. and needs your help falling back to sleep for another few hours. Instead, the lark is one who jumps out of bed at 5 A.M., eager to start her day—and insistent that you start yours as well. If you've got a lark, you need to move her sleep schedule backward, so that she falls asleep later in the evening, perhaps at 8 P.M., and stays in bed until 7 A.M.

First, get light to work in your favor. "Keep rooms very brightly lit in the evening, to help her stay awake longer," Dr. Sheldon suggests. "Also, hang heavy draperies or shades in her bedroom, to block out the early-morning sun. This may help her sleep later. . . ."

Some early risers can be taught to play alone quietly for half an hour or more, so their parents can catch an extra forty winks. Place some soft toys and cloth books in her crib the night before (but none large enough for the child to stand on and climb out). For a youngster already in a big bed, prepare a "bed box" of special playthings to be used only when the child awakes in the morning. Dr. Schmitt's suggestion: Buy her a clock radio, and establish a new rule that she must play quietly in her own room until the music comes on. . . .

From the Editors of **child** Magazine

SLEEP

how to teach
your child to sleep
like a baby

Tamara Eberlein

A New Century Communications Book

POCKET BOOKS

New York   London   Toronto   Sydney   Tokyo   Singapore

The author of this book is not a physician and the ideas, procedures, and suggestions in this book are not intended as a substitute for the medical advice of a trained health professional. All matters regarding your child's health require medical supervision. Consult your child's physician before adopting the suggestions in this book, as well as about any condition that may require diagnosis or medical attention. The author and publisher disclaim any liability arising directly or indirectly from the use of the book.

An *Original* Publication of POCKET BOOKS

POCKET BOOKS, a division of Simon & Schuster Inc.
1230 Avenue of the Americas, New York, NY 10020

Copyright © 1996 by Peggy Schmidt

All rights reserved, including the right to reproduce this book or portions thereof in any form whatsoever. For information address Pocket Books, 1230 Avenue of the Americas, New York, NY 10020

ISBN: 0-671-88038-1

First Pocket Books printing July 1996

10 9 8 7 6 5 4 3 2 1

POCKET and colophon are registered trademarks of Simon & Schuster Inc.

Cover photo by Tosca Radigonda Felicello

Printed in the U.S.A.

To my husband,
Bill Garvey,
and the children we cherish:
Michael,
James,
Samantha,
and Jack

Acknowledgments

Without the generous assistance of many people, this book could not have been written. I offer sincere thanks in particular to the following health-care professionals, who freely shared their time and expertise in the course of lengthy interviews:

T. Berry Brazelton, M.D., clinical professor of pediatrics emeritus at Harvard Medical School, professor of pediatrics and human development at Brown University, and author of *Touchpoints*

Lee J. Brooks, M.D., director of the Sleep Disorder Center at Rainbow Babies and Children's Hospital, and assistant professor of pediatrics at Case Western Reserve University in Cleveland

Elizabeth M. Bryan, M.D., pediatrician and medical director of the Multiple Births Foundation in London, and author of *Twins, Triplets and More*

Mary A. Carskadon, Ph.D., director of chronobiology at E. P. Bradley Hospital, and professor of psychiatry and human behavior at Brown University in Providence, Rhode Island

Ronald E. Dahl, M.D., director of the Child and Adolescent Sleep Laboratory at the Western Psychiatric Institute and Clinic in Pittsburgh and associate professor of pediatrics and psychiatry at the University of Pittsburgh Medical School

Richard Ferber, M.D., director of the Center for Pediatric Sleep Disorders at Children's Hospital in Boston, assistant professor of neurology at Harvard Medical School in Cambridge, Massachusetts, and author of *Solve Your Child's Sleep Problems*

Tiffany Field, Ph.D., professor of psychology, pediatrics, and psychiatry at the University of Miami School of Medicine, and director of the Touch Research Institute

May Griebel, M.D., codirector of the Sleep Disorders Center at Arkansas Children's Hospital in Little Rock, and assistant professor of pediatrics and neurology at the University of Arkansas for Medical Sciences

Jessie R. Groothuis, M.D., professor of pediatrics at the University of Colorado School of Medicine and the Children's Hospital in Denver

John Herman, Ph.D., director of the Sleep Disorders Center for Children at Children's Medical Center in Dallas

Penelope Leach, Ph.D., British psychologist and author of *Your Baby & Child from Birth to Age Five*

Alexander K. C. Leung, M.D., clinical associate professor of pediatrics at the University of Calgary in Alberta, Canada

Deborah Madansky, M.D., associate professor of

pediatrics and psychiatry at the University of Massachusetts Medical Center in Worcester

James McKenna, Ph.D., professor of anthropology at Pomona College in Claremont, California

Jodi A. Mindell, Ph.D., pediatric clinical psychologist for the Sleep Disorders Center and assistant professor of neurology at the Medical College of Pennsylvania, and assistant professor of psychology at St. Joseph's University in Philadelphia

Joseph Neidhardt, M.D., nightmare researcher in New Mexico and coauthor of *Conquering Bad Dreams and Nightmares*

Vaughn I. Rickert, Psy.D., pediatric psychologist and associate professor of pediatrics at the University of Arkansas for Medical Sciences in Little Rock

Charles E. Schaefer, Ph.D., director of the Better Sleep Center and professor of psychology at Fairleigh Dickinson University in Hackensack, New Jersey, and coauthor of *Winning Bedtime Battles* and *Raising Baby Right*

Martin Scharf, Ph.D., director of the Center for Research in Sleep Disorders at Mercy Hospital in Cincinnati, and author of *Waking Up Dry: How to End Bedwetting Forever*

Barton D. Schmitt, M.D., director of general pediatric consultative services at Children's Hospital of Denver, professor of pediatrics at the University of Colorado School of Medicine, and author of *Your Child's Health*

Deborah E. Sewitch, Ph.D., director of the Sleep-Wake Disorders Center at Hampstead Hospital in Hampstead, New Hampshire

Stephen Sheldon, D.O., director of the Center for Pediatric Sleep Medicine at Grant Hospital in Chicago, and clinical associate professor of pediatrics at the University of Chicago

Benjamin Spock, M.D., pediatrician and author of *Baby and Child Care*

Michael Stevenson, Ph.D., clinical director of the North Valley Sleep Disorders Center in Mission Hills, California

Michael Thorpy, M.D., director of the Sleep-Wake Disorders Center at Montefiore Medical Center in the Bronx, New York

Amy Wolfson, Ph.D., senior research associate at the E. P. Bradley Hospital Sleep Research Laboratory in Providence, Rhode Island, and assistant professor of psychology at College of the Holy Cross in Worcester, Massachusetts

Many thanks also to my tireless and inspiring editors, Peggy Schmidt of New Century Communications, Pamela Abrams of *Child* magazine, and Claire Zion of Pocket Books.

A big hug to my children, James, Samantha, and Jack Garvey, who waited patiently and sacrificed much playtime while Mommy was writing. And a very special thank-you to my husband, William Garvey, for his invaluable editorial counsel and unwavering emotional support.

Contents

Letter from the Editor

Dear Reader:

Expectant parents are quick to fill their shelves with books to prepare them for what's to come. But once the baby arrives, moms and dads are more likely to turn to information that's accessible, to the point, and a quick read. We created the *Child* Magazine Series for Parents for just that reason.

What makes the *Child* Magazine Series for Parents unique is that each book is intended to help parents of young children—babies, toddlers, preschoolers, and early school-age children—deal with a specific problem—quickly. The books are written by accomplished journalists who have picked the brains of leading child psychologists, researchers, and child-care experts and organized their collective wisdom. The benefit to you is that you will be presented with a number of strategies for understanding and coping with your child's behavior. You can select the one that best suits your parenting style, or try more than one if the first one you choose doesn't achieve the change you're looking for.

If you're a busy parent who needs help *now* to solve the problem featured in this book, I hope you will pick it up and start reading it tonight. I'm sure that the small investment of your time will provide a quick return as you implement the solutions we present. Throughout the book, you will find age "flags" that will help you easily find the sections that relate most directly to your situation. And if you find this advice helpful, try another book in this series; each one is written in the same friendly, informative style as *Child* magazine articles.

We'd love to hear from you after you have read the book. Let us know what worked for you, and whether you have any additional ideas that we might include in future editions of this book. Write to us at: *Child, Child Magazine Series for Parents,* 110 Fifth Avenue, New York, NY 10003. Or e-mail us at: Childmag@aol.com.

Pamela Abrams
Editor-in-Chief

Introduction

I'd Give Anything for a Good Night's Sleep

The crying woke me. Groaning, I glanced at the clock: 1 A.M. I'd stayed up late to help my mother prepare for the following day's family reunion, and hadn't made my way to her guest room until after midnight.

Groggily, I got out of bed, stumbled across the room to the portable crib where my 10-week-old son James was howling, and picked him up. Nursing, he calmed down and soon slept again. I eased him back to bed and climbed gratefully under my covers. But just as I started to slip into sleep, there came another cry—from James's twin sister, Samantha. As I sat on the bed nursing her, my eyes closed, my head nodded, and my body went limp. Suddenly I came to with a jerk, realizing with horror that the baby was falling out of my arms. Shocked but unhurt, Samantha started to wail—and James, waking again, mingled his screams with hers.

I could barely keep from screaming myself. Instead, I burst into tears, put my hands over my ears, and begged my babies to be quiet. They cried louder. In desperation, I scooped them both up and staggered downstairs to the kitchen where Mom was still at work. "You've got to take them for a while," I sobbed. "I can't stand it anymore. I haven't slept in weeks, and I'm so tired. If I don't get some rest, I'm going to throw myself out a window!"

If you're a parent, you're probably all too familiar with that feeling—because when kids don't sleep well, Mom and Dad don't either. That can lead to a plethora of problems, since sleep deprivation can affect every facet of your life.

If you're a mother who also works outside the home, you are practically guaranteed to be sleep deprived. According to the National Commission on Sleep Disorders Research, the average American has added 158 more hours per year to the work schedule since 1969—and for working mothers, the increase has been 241 hours.

The Effects of Sleep Deprivation on Adults

Brain power is often the first to go. Studies show that lack of sleep impairs memory, reasoning, concentration, speech, and decision making. Marey Oakes can attest to that: "My second daughter, Grace, didn't sleep through the night till she was nearly a year old, so for months I was utterly exhausted. I found myself doing things I normally never would do, like bouncing checks and misplacing things. I'd put the milk in the pantry and my eyeglasses in the refrigerator, then having to hunt for hours before finding them."

When we don't get enough sleep, we start to accumulate a sleep debt or sleep deficit. This represents the amount of sleep we needed but didn't get. Because it's cumulative, missing out on even an hour or two of rest each night means we wind up, after a few days, with a serious sleep deficit. And this debt must be paid back, either by staying in bed late on Saturday morning, dozing during play group, or, tragically, falling asleep behind the wheel. In fact, surveys from the Department of Transportation suggest that as many as 10 percent of traffic accidents are sleep related. Marey almost had one happen: "I was driving down the highway and couldn't summon the energy to flip on my turn signal or even look to the side before starting to change lanes. I was almost run down by an 18-wheeler."

When our kids' poor sleep habits rob us of rest, we also may become more prone to illness. For example, researchers have found that certain immune-system activity decreases as much as 30 percent on those nights when people miss three hours of sleep or more.

Sleep Problems Can Lead to Marital Discord

Mental health suffers as well. Studies show that depression among parents often is related to the severity of their children's sleep disturbances, according to Jodi A. Mindell, Ph.D., pediatric clinical psychologist for the Sleep Disorders Center at the Medical College of Pennsylvania in Philadelphia. Kids' sleep problems can cause conflicts between couples, too. "Parents whose children sleep poorly are far more likely to experience marital dissatisfaction," says Dr. Mindell. "I've seen many couples get to the brink of divorce over this."

Brett Holmes (not her real name) has a two-year-old son with multiple sleep problems. "It's been terrible to see how exhaustion has affected our marriage. We always had a great relationship, but now we snap at each other constantly. As for sex, forget it—we're too tired, and even when we're not, we don't feel friendly enough to make love. My husband and I have been through a lot together, but this problem is tearing us apart."

One reason relationships suffer in such circumstances is that couples "are robbed of private time that serves to restore the parents' emotional strength and sanity," notes Charles E. Schaefer, Ph.D., director of the Better Sleep Center at Fairleigh Dickinson University in Hackensack, New Jersey. Betsy Robinson (not her real name), a mother of two, laments, "Our 11-month-old demands so much attention at night that my husband and I have to take turns being 'on duty.' One of us stays upstairs in the guest room next to the nursery, while the other sleeps in the master bedroom downstairs. This has gone on for months. My husband and I never see each other. We're starting to wonder, 'Who is this person? Why did we get married?'"

Tensions run particularly high when partners disagree on how to handle the situation. Mom Audrey Cope confesses, "Sometimes our baby would be crying at night and I'd want to run to him. But Bruce would hold me there in bed, insisting that we let William cry so he'd learn to go back to sleep on his own. We had some huge fights about this."

The marital relationship is not the only one that suffers when parents are sleep deprived; so does the relationship between parent and child. No wonder, says Dr. Mindell: "After a rough night punctuated by tearful pleading or angry power struggles, it's hard to be enthusiastic about seeing your child again in the morning." With a catch in her voice, Betsy Robinson admits, "I love my son, but I also resent him. I feel frustrated, irritable, and impatient with him."

Sleep Problems Can Affect Kids' Health and Well-Being, Too

Bad as all this is, many loving parents say they're willing to sacrifice their own well-being and put up with their youngster's disruptive sleep habits, if doing so is in the best interests of the child. But the fact is, this is not in the best interests of the child. "During deep sleep, a youngster's body secretes hormones necessary for growth. Chronic sleep problems can inhibit this process, interfering with physical development," explains Martin Scharf, Ph.D., director of the Center for Research in Sleep Disorders at Mercy Hospital in Cincinnati. And like adults, sleep-deprived kids are more prone to accidents.

Children suffering from a lack of sleep also show signs of intellectual impairment, such as poor concentration, poor memory, and loss of creativity. They may feel extremely anxious, and have problems developing independence and self-confidence. What's more, chronic overtiredness can cause a variety of behavioral problems—aggression, irritability, defiance, lack of cooperation, and inability to tolerate frustration. "Parents may begin to blame a child for such behaviors, when in fact these are symptoms of an inappropriate amount of sleep," says Harvard Medical School professor Richard Ferber, M.D., director of the Center for Pediatric Sleep Disorders at Children's Hospital in Boston.

Just what are sleep problems? They're not the erratic sleep schedules and frequent nighttime wakings of newborns; these are normal and to be expected. Ideas on how to minimize the disruption that an infant's sleep cause you are, however, discussed in this book. Sleep problems arise when infantile sleep patterns persist too long, or new bad habits form as the child moves into toddlerhood and beyond.

Feel selfish for wanting a good night's sleep? You're not alone. "When it comes to helping kids establish good sleep habits, parents feel guilty for forcing the issue. Yet they needn't," says sleep researcher Amy Wolfson, Ph.D., assistant professor of psychology at College of the Holy Cross in Worcester, Massachusetts. "Think of it this way: no matter how much a youngster complains or begs, you wouldn't let him eat only sweets or spend the whole day watching TV. Adequate sleep is just as important to your youngster's well-being as a healthful diet and appropriate intellectual stimulation."

This book can help you solve your child's sleep problems and, in the process, your own. Chapter One gives guidelines on how much sleep a child needs at various ages. It will also help you determine whether your youngster is sleep deprived and outlines appropriate bedtime and naptime schedules. Chapter Two offers advice on how to handle a child who cries, complains, protests, or procrastinates at bedtime. In Chapter Three, there are strategies to put an end to those exhausting middle-of-the-night awakenings, when a child insists on having food, fun, or comforting. Chapter Four deals with night frights of various types: separation anxiety, phobias, nightmares, and night terrors. Chapter Five addresses the decision of whether to make your bed a family bed. It also discusses the important issue of where a child should sleep at different ages—in a bassinet, crib, big-kid bed—and explores various options for eliciting the child's cooperation. Finally, Chapter Six covers special sleep situations you may have trouble finding information on elsewhere, and also explains sleep disorders that may require professional help.

The information and advice in these chapters is based on in-depth interviews with more than two dozen of today's leading experts in sleep research, pediatric medicine, and child psychology, as well as thorough review of the existing literature on the subject of sleep problems. (For a complete list of experts, please see Acknowledgments on pages vii–x; for books and magazine articles, see Resources on pages 211–14.) Also featured are stories and hard-earned insights from more than 30 parents who have struggled with the same problems you're now facing.

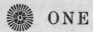 ONE

*Understanding Your
Child's Sleep Patterns
and Problems*

As many as 50 percent of children under the age of 6 have some type of bedtime problem, estimates the National Sleep Foundation. Why so many? Because a great number of parents don't know how to prevent such problems, or how to solve them when they do arise. Nor are parents sure where to turn for help. "Often the advice offered by pediatricians—changing the child's diet or feeding schedule, giving sedatives, or suggesting that parents simply wait for the child to outgrow the problem—are not effective," says Jodi A. Mindell, Ph.D., pediatric clinical psychologist for the Sleep Disorders Center at the Medical College of Pennsylvania in Philadelphia.

Even if they've been given good counsel on sleep training, parents may find reasons to delay acting on it. Betsy Robinson explains, "As an infant, Nicholas had bad colic and troublesome food sensitivities, so my husband and I didn't feel right about letting him cry, even when we knew it was time for him to sleep. Once he reached 8 months, we figured he was old enough to learn to sleep through the night. But then he started to cut teeth, and I couldn't leave him crying in his crib when he was in pain. Now he's 11 months old and still wakes up three times every night. Yet with winter coming, I know he'll catch colds from his big brother, and that will make it harder for him to sleep. Maybe I'll just wait till the spring to see if he starts sleeping through the night on his own."

Unfortunately for Betsy, this is probably wishful thinking. Studies show that spontaneous resolution of sleep problems is unlikely in over 80 percent of all children, according to Dr. Mindell. In fact, problems typically become more difficult to correct as the child gets older. Bad habits become more firmly entrenched, and the child struggles harder against whatever measures parents take to correct the situation.

But don't despair if you've let things go on longer than they should. "Most common sleep problems among infants and young children can be easily resolved in a week or two—sometimes sooner—if parents change their tactics," says Barton D. Schmitt, M.D., a specialist in behavioral pediatrics at the University of Colorado School of Medicine in Denver.

Admittedly, sleep training can be tough going at the start. "During the first 3 to 7 days of treatment, children generally take even longer to fall asleep at bedtime, or to fall back to sleep after waking in the middle of the night. But very soon, as the child adjusts to the new routine, she will fall asleep much quicker than she did before," says Dr. Mindell in assurance.

Tempted to give up and give in during that first difficult night of sleep training? Hang in there. "You may feel like the disruption caused by some of the methods is worse than the disruption caused by the sleep problem itself," says Deborah Madansky, M.D., associate professor of pediatrics and psychiatry at the University of Massachusetts Medical Center in Worcester. "But most problems will improve quickly. A week of disruption is not a high price to pay for a long-term solution."

Finding that solution, however, can be challenging. There's no universal panacea, no one "right" solution to children's sleep problems—only solutions that feel right to an individual parent. "Methods used must conform to a parent's own ideas about good child rearing, to the particular child's age and personality, and to the unique needs of that family," explains Dr. Madansky. "There's no such thing as a one-size-fits-all technique."

That's why this book presents a variety of options—some of which may even be contradictory—for handling sleep problems. Try those that seem most sensible and appropriate to you. But before you begin, discuss the various options with your partner, and try to reach an agreement on the best way to approach the problem. Otherwise, your chances of success are greatly reduced.

"If there's any rift between mother and father, the child will play that rift for all it's worth," cautions John Herman, Ph.D., director of the Sleep Disorders Center for Children, at Children's Medical Center in Dallas. "Suppose a child whines that he wants to sleep with his parents. Dad says no, but Mom says, 'Oh, let him in. It's the only way he'll get any sleep.' So the child crawls in next to Mommy. But it's a Pyrrhic victory for him; he doesn't really feel good about winning that battle. He knows he's angered his father and caused conflict between his parents, so he doesn't sleep well. And neither do Mom and Dad."

Once you have selected a method, give it time to work. Prematurely abandoning a technique not only ruins your chances for success with that method, but it can also make it more difficult to succeed with subsequent methods. Dr. Herman explains, "If you establish a new rule but then later give in to the child, this sets up what psychologists call a 'random reinforcement schedule.' The child learns only that if he complains enough, sometimes you will give in. So he keeps on complaining every night, hoping that tonight will be one of the 'lucky' nights in which he wins the conflict. Behavior motivated by a random reinforcement schedule is the most difficult type of behavior to modify. That's why it's best not to even start treating a sleep problem until you are completely committed to not falling back into your old patterns."

This isn't to say you need to stick with an unsuccessful method forever. A good rule of thumb: carefully select a method, use it faithfully for 2 weeks; if you see no signs of progress, try another tactic.

A Primer on the Science of Sleep

Before you try to change your child's sleep habits, it's helpful to know a bit about the physiology of sleep. There are two distinct types of sleep, REM (which stands for rapid eye movement) and non-REM. A person starts the night with non-REM sleep, which is divided into four stages: drowsiness, light sleep, deep sleep, and very deep sleep. During non-REM sleep, the heart beats slowly and regularly, breathing is slow and even, and there is little movement. The body and brain rest and recover from the rigors of the day. Typically, a person goes through one or two cycles of the non-REM stages, which takes about one to two hours, then makes the transition to REM sleep.

During REM sleep, a person may move about, his face muscles twitch, his eyes move rapidly under the closed lids, and his heartbeat and breathing are somewhat irregular. The mind is very active; this is when dreaming occurs. REM typically lasts from 10 to 40 minutes. While no one knows for sure what purpose REM sleep serves, some researchers speculate that it may help us absorb and interpret the events of our waking hours.

Typically, we go back and forth between non-REM and REM sleep perhaps half a dozen times every night, with each non-REM cycle becoming progressively lighter and each REM cycle progressively longer. When we complete the number of sleep cycles we require, we arise feeling rested and refreshed.

No matter how soundly we have slept, however, our sleep was not continuous and unbroken. Remember this: everyone wakes up spontaneously several times a night. (We discuss the vital significance of this fact in Chapter Three.) These wakings, which are usually brief and often forgotten, are a function of normal sleep cycles; they occur as we make the transition from one phase of sleep to another.

Adult Symptoms of Sleep Deprivation

* You need an alarm clock to wake up in the morning.
* On those mornings when the kids don't wake you, you sleep in for several hours.
* You need caffeine to remain alert.
* You often wish you could be taking a nap rather than doing whatever you're doing.
* You get sleepy when you drive for an hour or so.
* You doze off while reading or watching TV.
* You often feel irritable with your spouse or children.

Children's Sleep Differs from Adults' Sleep

Children's sleep differs from that of adults in several ways. For one thing, a very young child goes into deep sleep faster. "A 9-month-old can be screaming one minute and asleep the next. And she can travel the path from light to deep sleep within 2 minutes, while for an adult this process takes about 10 minutes," explains Richard Ferber, M.D., director of the Center for Pediatric Sleep Disorders at Children's Hospital in Boston. (The importance of this will become clear as we move ahead to Chapter Two.)

Little people also spend a greater percentage of their sleep time in REM. A newborn's sleep is about half REM; a toddler's sleep is one-third REM; by adulthood, REM comprises only one-fourth of total sleep time. In part, this accounts for the fact that children move around much more during sleep than do adults, since REM is a more active phase than non-REM. It's not uncommon to find a child, a few hours after bedtime, with his head against the footboard and his feet dangling off the edge of the mattress. Such contortions don't mean a child is unduly agitated; he's just sleeping like a, well, baby.

AGE FLAG: 3 TO 5 YEARS

Despite this twisting and turning, youngsters sleep far more deeply than adults do. When in very deep (stage four) sleep, a child is quite unresponsive to sound, light, movement, and other stimuli; at this time, he is almost impossible to rouse. It's during this stage that you can carry your sleeping child from the car into the house, change his diaper or place him on the toilet, put on his pajamas, and tuck him into bed—all without really waking him. "The amount and intensity of deep sleep appear to reach a developmental peak in the preschool years, and may be related to a child's giving up daytime naps," says Mary A. Carskadon, Ph.D., director of chronobiology at E. P. Bradley Hospital in Providence, Rhode Island.

AGE FLAG: 6 MONTHS AND UP

Another unique aspect is that children are more prone to enter a "mixed" state of sleep and arousal, in which they are neither completely asleep nor completely awake. These partial awakenings occur as a child makes the transition from one sleep phase to another, and his brain wave activity changes abruptly. The child may move about, change positions, rub his face, blink, whimper, or mumble before settling down again. Or he may experience an episode of night terrors (discussed in Chapter Four) or sleepwalking (explained in Chapter Six).

INFANTS ONLY: MAKING SENSE OF YOUR NEWBORN'S SLEEP

Physiologically, an infant's slumber differs somewhat from that of an older child. "When speaking of sleep in infants, we use different language. Instead of non-REM and REM, we talk about 'quiet sleep' and 'active sleep,'" says Dr. Carskadon. Even before birth, by the eighth month of pregnancy or earlier, a baby's sleep periods consist of these same two distinct phases.

Quiet sleep is characterized by limited movement, little brain activity, and slow eye movement. During active sleep, however, an infant may groan and sigh, move her eyes, suck, smile, jerk her arms and legs, and turn 360 degrees or more. Why so? Dr. Ferber explains, "During sleep, a person's brain sends frequent signals telling the various muscles of the body to move. In adults, these signals are blocked in the spinal cord so the sleeper is virtually paralyzed. But in infants, this blocking mechanism is not yet mature, so more signals get through to the muscles."

Making such twists and turns even more noticeable is the fact that—unlike an adult, who upon dropping off enters first into restful non-REM repose—a newborn plunges straight into active sleep. This gives parents ample opportunity to observe all those grunts and twitches before they close the nursery door.

For parents unaware of this phenomenon, the sight of their baby in active sleep can be a disconcerting one, adds May Griebel, M.D., codirector of the Sleep

Disorders Center at Arkansas Children's Hospital in Little Rock. "Parents sometimes think these intermittent twitches are symptoms of a seizure. But this is just normal active sleep. Unless the baby's twitching is rhythmic, constant, and prolonged, there's no need to worry," she says.

HOW MUCH IS A KID SUPPOSED TO SLEEP, ANYWAY?

There's no easy answer to the question of how much sleep a child should get. An individual child's need for sleep is affected not only by her age, but also by personality, biological patterns, rate of development, level of physical activity, health, emotional state, and environment. Nevertheless, by comparing how much your child sleeps to the table of average sleep needs below, you can tell if your youngster's in the ballpark for his or her age.

AVERAGE SLEEP NEEDS BASED ON AGE (IN HOURS)

Child's Age	Daytime Napping	Nighttime Sleep	Total in 24-Hour Period
1 week	8	8½	16½
1 month	7	8½	15½
3 months	5	10	15
6 months	4	10½	14½
9 months	3	11	14
1 year	2½	11½	14
1½ years	2	11½	13½

Child's Age	Daytime Napping	Nighttime Sleep	Total in 24-Hour Period
2 years	1½	11½	13
3 years	1	11	12
4 years		11½	11½
5 years		11	11

When your child sleeps less than you think he should, it could be that he simply needs less sleep than the typical child. Statistics such as those in the preceding table are only averages; they conceal a wide range of individual differences. A person's sleep needs can vary substantially from the average without falling outside the realm of normal. "A child's level of alertness during the day is a good indicator of whether he's getting enough sleep," explains Deborah E. Sewitch, Ph.D., director of the Sleep-Wake Disorders Center of Hampstead Hospital in Hampstead, New Hampshire. As long as he wakes up feeling refreshed and maintains a reasonable energy level until it's time for bed again, he's probably getting enough rest.

Or perhaps you're underestimating the amount of time your child spends sleeping. This is especially easy to do with babies, since they sleep in shorter, often unpredictable chunks of time rather than in long, solid blocks.

Consider, too, the possibility that your child's sleep quota is close to the average, but that this amount of slumber is less than you might find convenient. "A parent who gets upset because a child doesn't stay in bed for many, many hours on end should consider the child's needs, not just her own convenience. If she puts a child to bed early so she can have her evenings free, she must be prepared for the child to wake up early, too. Or if she wants to sleep late in the mornings, she'll have to let the child stay up longer at night," notes Dr. Ferber.

Signs of Chronic Sleep Debt in Children

* Difficult to awaken in the morning
* Sleeps late on weekends
* Frequently irritable, cranky, argumentative
* Often inattentive, impulsive, easily frustrated
* Often falls asleep during playtime at daycare or school, or before or during dinner
* Rubs his or her eyes; has droopy eyes

Determining whether your child is getting enough sleep means paying close attention to signs of sleep debt. Robin Hardin, a mother of three, describes how she made that diagnosis with her middle child. "Our problem started when Nikki entered kindergarten and had to start getting up for school. I think she goes to bed at a reasonable time and sleeps about as much as her older sister did at this age—yet she's impossible to wake up in the morning. At 7 A.M., I turn on the lights in her room and raise the blinds, then carry her into the bathroom. I set her down so she's forced to wake up enough to walk across the room to the toilet. If I don't go through this routine, then by the time I've woken up the other kids and gone back to check on Nikki, she has gone back to sleep." The clincher: Nikki always stays in bed until 10 A.M. on weekends and school holidays.

There is one other sign of sleep deprivation in children that is quite common yet is frequently misinterpreted: hyperactivity. "It's easy to be fooled into thinking that a high level of late-evening activity indicates your child has a reserve of energy that needs to be expended. But being overtired can trigger the release of stimulating chemicals, adrenaline and noradrenaline, that fight fatigue. This can make the child seem wide awake and revved up—she may be jumping all around the room at 10 P.M.—even though what she most needs is sleep," explains Charles E. Schaefer, Ph.D., director of the Better Sleep Center at Fairleigh Dickinson University in Hackensack, New Jersey.

AGE FLAG: 9 MONTHS AND UP

You're unlikely to observe this paradoxical behavior in an infant; typically, babies sleep when they are tired, no matter where or when. Yet by the time a child is 9 months old, he may start to get so wired that he simply cannot relax enough to go to sleep. "In a toddler, excitement and tension can build up to the point where he no longer knows that he is tired, does not see how to stop and rest, and cannot relax anyway," says British psychologist Penelope Leach, Ph.D. "Look at what he is doing and see whether he is finding it more difficult than he did half an hour ago. If he is, then he needs a rest." Although it may take a couple weeks for the beneficial effects to become noticeable, once such a "hyper" child starts to get a more appropriate amount of sleep, he's likely to be calmer during the day, have improved self-control, and show normal signs of weariness in the evening.

INFANTS ONLY: DO YOU THINK YOUR NEWBORN SLEEPS TOO LITTLE—OR TOO MUCH?

If you have a newborn, it's not accurate or even fair to refer to her frequent round-the-clock awakenings as a "sleep problem." She's just doing what virtually all infants do to ensure that they receive the near-constant nourishment they need. But those multiple middle-of-the-night wakings certainly can be a problem for you, as unbroken blocks of sleep become but a distant memory, desperately missed.

To help you put your mind (if not your weary body) to rest, remember this: in the early weeks, there's no trick to knowing whether your child is sleeping too much or too little. He isn't doing either. "A baby will get all the sleep he requires, as long as he's not hungry, uncomfortable, or constantly interrupted. He cannot resist the urge to sleep when he's tired, nor can he keep on sleeping when no longer tired," explains Amy Wolfson, Ph.D., assistant professor of psychology at College of the Holy Cross in Worcester, Massachusetts.

While the table presented earlier lists the average sleep time for a newborn as 16½ hours in a 24-hour period, studies show that a particular infant may sleep as little as 10 hours or as much as 22 hours. If your baby falls on the short side of normal, there's not much you can do about it other than lower your expectations for how much you're going to accomplish "while the baby naps." Console yourself with the thought that your active infant may be more fun to play with than a baby who sleeps the day away. And be prepared to start now to find a pattern in your infant's seemingly patternless and extra-short sleep, and build on it. (See Chapter Three for details.)

What if your newborn is just the opposite? Not to worry. "As an infant, my youngest daughter did nothing but eat and sleep. It seemed she was out cold 20 hours a day. I started to get worried," says Lisa Cool, a mother of three. Lisa voiced her concerns to her pediatrician. "He laughed and said that I was the first parent to complain that her baby slept too much. So I decided to relax and count myself lucky."

How a Sleep Log Can Help

One of the most worthwhile things you can do as you prepare to tackle a sleep problem is to keep a sleep log. Complete the log daily, recording the following information:

* Times at which the child appears to become sleepy
* Time and length of any naps
* Time at which the child is put to bed in the evening, and (as closely as you can determine) the time at which he or she actually falls asleep
* Times of any nighttime wakings, and how long the child stays awake

- Time the child awakes in the morning
- Child's total sleep time during that 24-hour period, calculated from the figures above
- Child's mood and energy level at various times during the day and evening
- Steps you take to get the child to sleep at naptime, bedtime, and after a night waking
- How long this process takes

At various points in this book, we discuss the importance of this diary to the success of certain methods used to treat specific sleep problems. For now, simply let the log help you get a handle on exactly what the problem is, so you can see more clearly what you need to change.

Why Consistency (with Bedtime) Matters

Some parents prefer not to establish a strict bedtime for their children, because they appreciate the freedom and spontaneity an unstructured schedule allows. Kirk Newhope (not his real name), the father of a 12-month-old, explains, "We like to pick up the baby and go whenever opportunity knocks. We don't worry that dinner with friends, or an 8 o'clock movie, or an evening trip to the mall is going to conflict with our daughter's bedtime."

For some families, this happy-go-lucky approach fits their lifestyle. But beware: there is usually a price to pay. Dr. Leach explains, "A baby who is kept up on occasion to suit your convenience is very unlikely to go happily to bed at a conventional hour just because that is what would suit you tonight. She will probably be the kind of toddler who is up until all hours most nights of the week, and whose daytime sleep pattern is also irregular."

Other parents avoid enforcing a regular bedtime, instead applying a policy of "let him run till he drops in his tracks." Their rationale is that, the more tired the child is at bedtime, the more soundly and longer he'll sleep. Unfortunately, this doesn't often pan out. "In many cases, if you wait until your child seems extremely sleepy before you put her to bed, you've waited too long. Being overtired is a form of stress, and when a person is stressed, her sleep suffers," says Dr. Schaefer. In such circumstances, a child is likely to have a very hard time falling asleep, or to experience more wakings during the night.

At the opposite end of the spectrum are those parents who strictly enforce bedtime, allowing very few exceptions. Lisa Cool is one such mom: "I am a firm believer in the wisdom of putting children to bed at the same time every evening. I pick a reasonable bedtime, then put my kids down at that time every night, no matter what. I find that the whole getting-to-sleep process goes much more smoothly if I don't vary the bedtime at all." Such a policy invites little argument from the kids, and ensures peace and privacy for parents in the evening. But there is a drawback. "This approach only works if it is kept to almost all the time," says Dr. Leach. "That means arranging your evenings out so that you put the baby to bed before you go, and having a babysitter. It means keeping as close to the normal pattern as you can even when you are on vacation, and arranging your trips to fit in with that routine."

Flexibility Is Fine . . . Within Certain Limits

You may find that you can be a bit flexible—letting kids stay up a little later when you have an out-of-town house guest, or designating Friday or Saturday as "late night"—without compromising kids' sleep requirements or cooperativeness. "But," Dr. Schaefer warns, "don't vary bedtime more than one night a week, and then not for more than one hour. Straying further from the routine could make a child more likely to want to stay up later at other times."

Amy Marz finds room for flexibility in her two preschoolers' schedule by clearly stating the limits: "If we are visiting Grandma or there's a special on TV, the girls can stay up an hour or so past their normal bedtime. But I'm always careful to cut the deal first, and make sure they understand it. I might say, 'Okay, you can watch all of *Mary Poppins*. But you must brush your teeth and put on your pajamas first, and as soon as the show's over, it's straight to bed.'"

Once your kids are accustomed to going to bed at a fairly regular time, think twice before succumbing to the temptation to keep them up late. They're almost sure to act out, as I learned one evening shortly before Halloween, when my twins were 4 and my younger son was 2. After a busy afternoon at preschool, I drove the kids to visit friends in our old hometown, a 45-minute drive. Then we attended a costume party, where all three stuffed themselves with candy corn and cupcakes in lieu of dinner. The party ended at 8:30—just the time I normally would have been tucking them all into bed. But instead of heading for home, I impulsively took them to visit yet another friend and her

3-year-old daughter, who lived nearby. Of course, the playdate was a disaster. My three whined, cried, fussed, and fought with their playmate for half an hour, until my friend's husband asked us to leave. I was humiliated and, at first, furious with my kids. But they were exhausted and passed out as soon as I buckled them into their carseats. I realized I had only myself to blame.

Selecting a Bedtime

Your next step is to pick a time at which you'll put your child to bed. This is not an arbitrary decision. If you select too early an hour, your child is likely to resist going to bed and, once under the covers, may lie awake a long time before falling asleep. If you delay bedtime until late, he may suffer the ill effects of sleep deprivation and fatigue-induced hyperactivity outlined earlier.

Start by taking some cues from your child. Your sleep log comes in handy here. How does his daytime mood and behavior change with the fluctuations in his bedtime? What time does he generally become tired in the evening? Learn your child's personal "sleepy signals"—rubbing his eyes or ears, sucking his thumb, being quick to cry, getting overly excited. Once you start watching for such signs, you'll spot them quickly. I still remember how easy it was to tell when my little brother Willy was tired; though he might still be charging around the room, his left eyelid would inevitably, uncontrollably, drop to half-mast.

Set bedtime for the hour at which your youngster typically becomes tired. Be prepared for some fine-tuning. If she takes an hour to drop off, yet wakes up in good spirits every day, push her bedtime back by 45 minutes or so. On the other hand, if she shows any signs of sleep deprivation, try putting her to bed earlier and see if the situation improves. Don't expect instant results—it may take 1 or 2 weeks for her internal clock to adjust to the change and for the benefits to become noticeable.

Enforcing the New Routine

AGE FLAG: 1 YEAR AND UP

Your next challenge is to persuade your child to adhere to the new routine. Here's a sample script of persuasive words, geared toward a preschooler, which you can adapt to your own situation. With toddlers, you may need to modify the words to suit the child's vocabulary, but many of the points made remain essentially the same. In Chapter Two, we'll go into more detail about the necessary rituals that precede going to sleep.

PARENT: Alex, it's 7:50. You may play with your blocks for 10 more minutes, until 8:00. Look, I'm setting the kitchen timer so when it rings, you'll know it's time to stop. Then I'll help you brush your teeth and put on your pajamas. We'll have all this done by 8:15—when the big hand is on the three and the little hand is on the eight—and then I'll read you a story. Then it's lights out at 8:30.

CHILD: I don't want to go to bed yet. I'm not sleepy.

PARENT: Remember how unpleasant you feel being dragged out of bed every morning? This new, earlier bedtime is to help you feel more cheerful and full of energy tomorrow.

CHILD: But Tim gets to stay up really late. You always let Tim do whatever he wants. It isn't fair.

PARENT: Tim has a bedtime, too. It's a little later than yours because he's older. Anyway, the rule is that you can play until 8:00, then we can read for a while. Tell you what: you can pick the story if you stop playing at 8:00.

CHILD: Okay. But what if I can't fall asleep once I'm in bed?

PARENT: You can take a few toy cars or some stuffed animals to bed with you, and play quietly until you feel sleepy.

CHILD: All right.

PARENT: (Hugs child.) Okay, sweetie. And thanks for cooperating.

This type of interaction accomplishes several things:

- It warns the child that bedtime is coming. Given a chance to finish his game, the child feels less resentful of the interruption bedtime represents.
- Using a timer—an impersonal signal—to indicate when it's time to begin the bedtime preparations helps reduce conflict between parent and child. "A child is less likely to argue against this kind of impersonal limit than against one that comes directly from you," explains Dr. Schaefer. If the child is old enough

to tell time, using the clock to signal bedtime can likewise limit struggles over authority.

- The parent clearly states what is expected of the child and the ways in which the parent will participate. The rules are phrased in a positive fashion—"you may play with your blocks for 10 more minutes," and "we can read for a while." Avoid negative phrasing, such as "you cannot stay up past 8:30," which makes bedtime feel like punishment.

- When challenged, the parent avoids a bossy response such as "It's bedtime now because I said so." Instead, she calmly gives a rational explanation for the rule. Your toddler's too young to understand the reason given above? To her you might simply say, "You must go to sleep now so you'll feel good tomorrow." Dr. Schaefer notes, "The child may not agree with your explanation, but at least he'll know that your new rules aren't arbitrary."

- Faced with further resistance from the child, the parent simply restates the rule rather than get drawn into a lengthy argument.

- Letting the child choose the bedtime story gives him a feeling of control, and so increases the likelihood that he'll cooperate. Likewise, you can let him select which pajamas to wear, which stuffed animals to take to bed, and which lullaby to sing.

- The parent uses positive reinforcement—a hug, a word of thanks—to acknowledge the child's cooperation. "Rewards are more effective motivators than penalties," notes Dr. Schaefer. You might also offer token tangible rewards such as stars on a chart, stickers, or even a small toy.

- By allowing the child to play quietly in his bed after

lights out, the parent acknowledges that she cannot force her son to fall asleep at a given time. Rather than insist that he lie in bed bored and frustrated while waiting for sleep to come, she establishes a situation in which the child can amuse himself while he winds down.

Working Parents and the Late-Bedtime Temptation

"I'm appalled at the thought of getting home from work at 7 P.M. and sending Maggie straight to bed. If I did, I'd never get to see her except on weekends," laments Gail Sheffler, creative director of a promotions agency and mother of a 3-year-old. "So we have dinner at 8:00, play till 9:15, and then get ready for bed. Maggie falls asleep around 10:00."

Maggie's not the only preschooler with a late lights-out. "We've noted a growing trend toward later bedtimes for kids, especially in single-parent and dual-career families, because parents want some quality time with their child once the workday is over," notes Dr. Carskadon. "Unfortunately, what often happens is that the child gets too little sleep. Parents wind up being unable to enjoy those evening hours devoted to family because the sleep-deprived child becomes irritable, contentious, and out of control."

Guilt may factor into the equation, too. A parent who feels conflicted about being away from the child all day may be less able to tolerate the protests that can accompany the establishment of a new, stricter bedtime policy. Thus, she may be more likely to give in to the child's whining, which only encourages the kid to rebel further. Indeed, a *Child* magazine survey found that mothers who work full time outside the home have 16 percent more trouble getting their kids to cooperate at bedtime than moms who work part time or stay at home.

AGE FLAG: 4 YEARS AND UNDER

Fortunately, there are ways to make a late bedtime work. "It's all right to put a child to bed late, provided she is able to sleep late in the morning," says Dr. Carskadon. This is quite manageable if you have a live-in nanny or a sitter who comes to your home each morning before you leave for work. If the child must wake early to go to daycare, an extra-long afternoon nap may leave room for an additional hour of family time in the evening. "Maggie has to get up at 8:45 3 days a week so the sitter can get her to preschool by 9:30, but the other days she sleeps in until 10 A.M.," explains Gail Sheffler.

If your youngster must get up early in the morning, and afternoon naps aren't solving the sleep-shortage problem, you have little choice but to put her to bed earlier. "Remind yourself that you and your child can have a wonderful time together, even if your evening interaction lasts only 45 minutes. Don't drag playtime out for 2 hours if that last hour is a disaster," urges Dr. Wolfson.

AGE FLAG: 5 YEARS AND UP

Even if your late-night routine is workable now, prepare yourself for the fact that it will have to change once your child starts school and is no longer able to sleep late or take naps. At that point, consider having the whole family go to bed earlier so you can all arise with the dawn and enjoy some early-morning togetherness before everyone heads off to work or school.

✷

How You Can Catch More Quality zzzz's

1. Nap when your baby naps. Baby's naptime may be your only chance to weed the garden or check in with the coworker who's filling in during your maternity leave, but sleep is more important. If possible, catch those 40 winks before 3 P.M. A later nap may make it more difficult for you to sleep well at night.

   Snoozing along with your infant is admittedly trickier if you also have an older child to take care of. To increase my odds of a successful siesta after the birth of my third child, I first babyproofed my family room to the nth degree. That done, I felt reasonably confident that my twins, then 2, could watch a video in safety while I dozed on the sofa next to them and the baby napped in the nursery.

2. Watch what you eat. Tempted to indulge in a midnight feast? Your stomach may become uncomfortably distended, and lying down will increase the likelihood of heartburn—neither of which promote restful repose. "It's also wise to avoid spicy meals late in the evening, since such fare can have a stimulant effect," notes Michael Thorpy, M.D., director of the Sleep-Wake Disorders Center at Montefiore Medical Center in the Bronx, New York. On the other hand, if you go to bed hungry, you may not be able to sleep as deeply. Trying to lose those pregnancy pounds? Save some of your day's allotted calories for a light bedtime snack.

3. Pay attention to your caffeine and alcohol intake. Try not to rely on coffee, tea, or cola to keep you alert; the caffeine these contain can make it harder for you to fall asleep when you want to. A good rule of thumb: consume no caffeine within 6 hours of bedtime—even more if you're especially sensitive to its effects. Watch your alcohol intake as well, and say no to after-dinner drinks. Dr. Thorpy explains, "Alcohol may make you feel sleepy initially, but later in the night it interferes with sleep quality. You are more likely to have nightmares, and you awaken feeling less refreshed."

4. Go to bed as early as you can. It's tempting to cram 10,000 tasks into those few hours that remain to you after the kids are in bed. But don't; you're better off hitting the hay yourself. Decide in advance what time to shut off the TV; if there's a good show on later, tape it on the VCR and watch it the next day. Schedule chores for weekend mornings. If you have a business trip, avoid scheduling any evening meetings; instead, seize the chance to go to bed early.

5. Schedule your workout for the morning or afternoon, not during evening hours. "Exercise triggers the release of adrenaline, which revs you up for several hours. If you work out too late in the day, you may have trouble falling asleep at bedtime," Dr. Thorpy explains.

6. Snooze when and where you can. Often when I'd take my three kids on an afternoon outing, they'd all fall asleep during the drive home. On such occasions, I'd turn off the car, crank back my seat, and nap in my driveway until someone awoke.

Or take a tip from Lisa McDonough: "My son was 4 and my daughter was 2 when I gave birth to boy/

girl twins. When my own birthday rolled around 2 months later, I told my husband that the best gift he could give me was a night in a luxury hotel. No, I wasn't dreaming about a romantic evening of fine wine and great food followed by fabulous sex. My ultimate fantasy was a night of uninterrupted sleep."

Stays Up Too Late? Wakes Up Too Early? How to Adjust a Child's Ill-Timed Sleep Schedule

At times a child's internal clock may fall out of sync with his family's daily schedule. He isn't sleep deprived—he's getting the right amount of rest—but he's getting it at the wrong time. This problem is known as a "sleep phase shift." Stephen Sheldon, D.O., director of the Center for Pediatric Sleep Medicine at Grant Hospital in Chicago, explains, "A youngster who tosses and turns and stares at the ceiling for several hours at bedtime and then is impossible to awaken in the morning may have a sleep-phase delay. A child who grows cranky and fatigued a few hours before bedtime but arises with the first rays of sun the next morning may have a sleep-phase advance."

Sleep-phase shifts can be quite problematic for parents. You may face countless bedtime battles each night, then have to drag the youngster away from his pillow in order to start your day. Or you may struggle with an overtired, short-tempered child at dinnertime, then be reluctantly forced from your own bed at dawn to take care of a wide-awake tot. Either way, it's not a happy situation. But fortunately, it's one you can change.

How to Handle a Night Owl

AGE FLAG: 6 MONTHS AND UP

In dealing with night owls, understand that we are not talking about a child who rebels against bedtime, nor one who is unable to get to sleep without endless ministrations from you. (These problems are covered in Chapter Two.) Rather, we're referring to a child who falls asleep peacefully, sleeps long and well, and wakes up cheerful if allowed to do so in his own good time—but does all this later than you wish him to. Your mission: to move his sleep schedule forward, so that he falls asleep earlier in the evening, and wakes up earlier the next morning.

The solution is not simply to set an early bedtime, warns Dr. Sheldon. "Suppose your child sleeps from 10 P.M. to 9 A.M., and you want him to sleep from 8 P.M. to 7 A.M. If you plop him in bed at 8:00, he'll lie awake for hours because he's not physiologically ready to sleep yet. This is not good. You want him to associate his bed with sleeping, not with staring into the dark feeling bored and frustrated."

Instead, you must gradually reset the child's internal clock. To start, use your sleep log to figure out how many hours your child sleeps when undisturbed, and the actual times she tends to drop off and wake up. Next, move her scheduled bedtime back to the hour she has actually been falling asleep. Don't worry; this 10 P.M. bedtime is only temporary. The second night, move her bedtime forward by 15 minutes—for example, to 9:45. After 1 week, move it forward another 15 minutes, to 9:30. Continue advancing the bedtime by a quarter of an hour each week, until eventually you

reach the desired 8 P.M. lights-out. "In children who
can't tell time, you can gradually—over 8 weeks or
so—achieve an 8 P.M. bedtime this way with very few
tantrums," says Dr. Schmitt.

Seems like a long, dragged-out process? You can
take a shortcut, if you're willing to put up with several
days of grouchiness. Dr. Sheldon explains, "To start,
let the child go to bed at whatever time he normally
falls asleep—for instance, 10 P.M. The next morning,
wake him at the time you want him to start getting
up—in this case, 7 A.M.—no matter how much he protests. That evening, he will be so tired that he'll fall
asleep earlier than usual, perhaps at 9:30. The following morning, wake him at 7 A.M. again. Within a few
days, if you're consistent about waking him at 7:00,
he should be falling asleep around 8:00."

Be prepared for battle in trying to get him out of
bed those first few days, since he most certainly won't
want to wake up. "Very bright lights may help, because light shuts off the secretion of the hormone mel-
atonin, thus signaling to the body that it is time to
wake up," says Dr. Sheldon. "Also, do schedule the
process for a time when the child has no social or
academic responsibilities, since he's bound to be tired
and irritable for a few days."

Once the new schedule is established, it's important
to continue being consistent with your wake-up call,
Dr. Sheldon warns. "If you let the child sleep in till 9
A.M. on weekends, his sleep phase will drift back toward the later position. He'll have a hard time falling
asleep Sunday night, and will be tough to awaken Mon-
day morning." If you feel he needs to sleep in occa-

sionally—following a late-night party, perhaps—be sure to rouse him no more than an hour past his new regular wake-up time.

With infants and toddlers, the slow-but-steady technique presented first is more effective because it is so difficult to keep a tired baby from falling back to sleep. The gradual approach also works for preschoolers and older kids, although by that point you may appreciate the quicker results of the second method. But note: whichever method you choose, you may also need to make some adjustments to the child's nap schedule. Naps are discussed later in this chapter.

How to Keep a Morning Lark Quiet a Bit Longer

A morning lark is not a child who wakes at 4 A.M. and needs your help falling back to sleep for another few hours. (This very disruptive problem is discussed in Chapter Three.) Instead, the lark is one who jumps out of bed at 5 A.M., eager to start her day—and insistent that you start yours as well. Yet by late afternoon, her energy's gone; she passes out at 6 P.M., leaving no opportunity for a family dinner or evening playtime with her parents. If you've got a lark, you need to move her sleep schedule backward, so that she falls asleep later in the evening, perhaps at 8 P.M., and stays in bed until 7 A.M.

First, get light to work in your favor. "Keep rooms very brightly lit in the evening, to help her stay awake longer," Dr. Sheldon suggests. "Also, hang heavy draperies or shades in her bedroom, to block out the early-morning sun. This may help her sleep later."

Next, let your activity level match the lighting. Instead of planting her in front of the TV in the early evening, where she's sure to fall asleep, play with her actively so she understands that staying awake at this time is fun and rewarding. Conversely, keep your early-morning activity to a minimum. The more boring you are at dawn, the more likely she is to find sleep an attractive alternative.

AGE FLAG: 9 MONTHS TO 2 YEARS

Some early risers can be taught to play alone quietly for half an hour or more, so their parents can catch an extra 40 winks. Place some soft toys and cloth books in her crib the night before (but none large enough for the child to stand on and climb out). Don't rush to her room at her first peep; give her a chance to learn to amuse herself.

AGE FLAG: 3 YEARS AND UP

For a youngster already in a big bed, prepare a "bed box" of special playthings—books, puzzles, audiotapes—to be used only when the child awakes in the morning. Dr. Schmitt's suggestion: buy her a clock radio, and establish a new rule that she must play quietly in her own room until the music comes on. Or do what Lisa Cool did with her early-bird twins when they were 4 years old: "I told them, 'When you wake up in the morning, look out the window. If it's still dark, try to go back to sleep or at least play quietly in your room. Once it gets light, you can come wake me up.'"

If the problem persists, you'll need to take a more active approach to adjusting the child's sleep phase. But there are no shortcuts. "Simply keeping the child up late for one or two nights does not help, because it does not allow enough time for the sleep phase to shift to a new time," explains Dr. Ferber. Instead, you must gradually change her bedtime and wake-up time—and you'll need to gradually change the schedule of her other daily activities as well.

Start by postponing meals and bedtime by 10 minutes. Suppose she normally eats breakfast at 5:30 A.M., begs for dinner at 5 P.M. (long before the rest of the family is ready to eat), and falls asleep at 6 P.M. The first day, feed her breakfast at 5:40 A.M., dinner at 5:10 P.M., and do whatever you can to keep her awake until 6:10. The next day, move everything back another 10 minutes, so she's not in bed until 6:20. Continue in this fashion until you've reached the desired bedtime. It should take about 12 days to achieve an 8 P.M. bedtime.

Will this later lights-out mean she'll sleep later in the morning? Yes—but probably not right away. "Often, the change in morning waking lags behind the other changes," Dr. Ferber observes. Yet within 3 weeks, the new schedule should be well established.

You may also need to adjust the child's naptime, particularly if she's one of those early risers who's ready for her morning nap an hour after breakfast. Kathleen Sweeney, a mother of two, found a solution: "When Max was 8 months old, he started getting up at 5 o'clock, and by 7 A.M., he was ready to nap. So after breakfast each morning, I strapped him into the backpack and took a long walk outside, where the fresh air and busy streets helped keep him awake. To postpone his afternoon nap, we played piggyback and other active games. Then in the evening, I gave him a big production of a bath, with his tape player blaring and tons of toys. My husband even climbed in the tub with him to make it more exciting. It took about a month, but it worked. We got his morning nap moved back to 10:30 A.M., his afternoon nap to 3:00, and his bedtime to 8:30. And the big payoff was that he slept each morning until about 7:30."

NAPS: HOW MANY, HOW LONG, WHEN TO STOP

When it comes to the number of naps taken daily, there are bound to be variations from day to day and from child to child. But knowing the averages can help you get a handle on whether or not your child's nap schedule is in line or out of whack with his age.

CHILD'S AGE	NUMBER OF NAPS DAILY
Newborn	4
1–6 months	3
6–18 months	2
18–36 months	1

If your child takes two or more naps a day, the length of those naps may be fairly equal, or they may be quite different. Some days it may seem that there's no predicting when he'll pass out. Yet the more consistent you can be with his schedule of daytime activities, the more likely it is he'll become sleepy and be willing to rest around the same time each day.

When Kids Nap Too Much

To busy parents desperate for a few hours of peace during the day, the idea that a child might nap too much may seem ludicrous. But it isn't—not if prolonged napping interferes with the child's ability to fall asleep at a reasonable hour of the evening, or stay asleep until a reasonable hour of the morning. Having a child who naps half the day away is no advantage if he then wants to stay up past midnight or awakens raring to go at 4:30 A.M.

If you suspect that overlong siestas are creating such problems, it would be wise to cut back on your child's daytime sleep. Start by limiting her afternoon nap to 1 to 2 hours at most. If the current routine does not leave at least 4 hours between the end of the nap and the child's regular bedtime, begin her nap earlier in the afternoon. "For children older than 1 year, naptime should be started early, by 1 P.M. Any nap after 3 P.M. will diminish the need for continuous and deep sleep during the night," explains child development expert T. Berry Brazelton, M.D., clinical professor of pediatrics emeritus at Harvard Medical School. If necessary, enlist the cooperation of your daycare provider in establishing the new schedule.

Waking a sleeping child is sometimes easier said than done (except, of course, at those times you do not want to awaken her, when the sound of dust falling seems to be sufficient to startle her into screaming consciousness). When you want to put an end to a nap, try going into her room and straightening up, or sing to her, or read aloud. This may avoid the angry outburst often produced by a child who has just been shaken awake. Don't scold him if he does wake up disoriented and irritable. Instead, offer him a snack or a cuddle, and soon he'll come around. "If you simply cannot rouse him no matter what you do, he's probably in a deep-sleep stage. Wait 15 minutes and then try again," adds Lee J. Brooks, M.D., director of the Sleep Disorder Center at Rainbow Babies and Children's Hospital in Cleveland, Ohio.

Making the Transition from Two Naps a Day to One

You should anticipate a difficult period sometime between the ages of 18 and 24 months, during which it will become evident that your child no longer requires two naps a day, yet one seems not quite enough. This can be a tricky transition, because you cannot simply drop one of the naps.

"Suppose your child has been napping at 10 A.M. and again at 2 P.M., yet seems ready to go to a single nap daily. If you just skip the morning nap, he'll fall asleep before you've had a chance to serve lunch. If you skip the afternoon nap, he'll never make it through till dinner without losing control," Dr. Wolfson explains.

"Instead, you need to adjust his entire daytime schedule. For example, you might play with him actively in the late morning to keep him awake from 10 to 11. Then give him an early lunch, and put him down for his nap around noon." Until the new routine is well established, try to be patient with the child's inevitable crankiness.

Naps No More

For most parents, it's a sad day when they realize their child no longer needs to nap at all. Gone is that daily respite from the rigors of child care, gone that luxurious hour during which you could phone a friend, fax your office, or finish a novel. It may happen abruptly, when a child suddenly refuses to nap at all. Or it may happen gradually, when a child sleeps some days but not others. However it happens, there's no doubt that it will happen; the only real question is when.

"Most kids stop napping sometime between the ages of 2 and 3, but there are 1-year-olds who refuse to take any naps, and 5-year-olds who still take a brief daytime nap," says Dr. Ferber. You cannot expect siblings to follow the same schedule on this. My twins napped until well past their third birthday, while their little brother Jack (much to my dismay) went on a permanent nap strike at 21 months.

With some careful observation, you should be able to tell when your child is ready to give up naps. Here again, your sleep log can help you keep track of your observations and guide you toward the right decision. Don't make it an arbitrary one; prematurely eliminating naptime can set the stage for nighttime sleep problems. Why? Because the child will feel tired in the afternoon, triggering the release of energy-boosting adrenaline. The resulting hyperactivity will make it hard for her to settle down at bedtime. She'll sleep poorly, and awake the next day feeling irritable and fatigued.

The following signs indicate that a child is not yet ready to stop napping:

- Slow to wake up in the morning
- Sleeps several hours later on weekend mornings
- Rubs eyes frequently
- Often seems drowsy; has little energy
- Is irritable and hard to control by late afternoon on the days he doesn't nap

On the other hand, a child who is ready to give up naps for good may show these signs:

- Sleeps less than 10 hours at night
- Takes an unusually long time to fall asleep at bedtime
- Often does not fall asleep at naptime, even if he stays in his bed
- Shows no undue signs of physical fatigue on no-nap days
- Is not particularly fussy or ill-behaved on the days he hasn't napped

What finally convinced me that my not-quite-2-year-old was a candidate for consolidating all his sleep at night? On the days I did coax him down for a nap, he'd lie in bed wide awake for hours that evening—and then sneak downstairs to watch the 11 o'clock nightly news. Giving up the nap got him back on track for an 8 P.M. bedtime.

Once you've made the decision to eliminate daytime

sleeping, consider replacing naptime with a regularly scheduled "quiet time." This makes the transition easier for you (since it allows you to retain your middle-of-the-day break) and for your child, who can use this rest period to restore physical energy and emotional equilibrium. "You can't force a child to sleep, but by establishing a regular quiet time, you help the child make a successful adjustment to no naps," says Dr. Schaefer.

Schedule quiet time for immediately after lunch, so you know the child isn't hungry. Lower the shades so it's not too bright, but leave enough light for him to see clearly. If you keep the house relatively quiet, he won't feel resentful about "missing out" on all the fascinating activities going on in his absence. Does your child continually pop out of his room to see what you're doing? It may help if you stay nearby (though not in his room) so he feels assured of your presence. Set the kitchen timer for 30 to 60 minutes to give him a sense of how long quiet time will last—and to avoid endless inquiries like "Is quiet time over yet?"

Keep the limits clear and simple: "It's quiet time now. You don't have to sleep, but you do have to stay quietly in your room for 45 minutes. You can look at books, play with puzzles, or color." You might bring out special toys that are available only during the rest period. Clare Gunther, a mother of two, offers another suggestion: "Since Anne knows how to operate her audiotape player by herself, I let her spend quiet time listening to music or storybook tapes. She knows that she can listen to as many as she wants, as long as she stays in her room."

What if the child does fall asleep during quiet time,

or later in the afternoon? "Wake him up after no more than 30 minutes," suggests Dr. Sheldon. "You can't let him sleep for an hour or two and then expect him to be able to settle down easily at bedtime." Plan for an adjustment period of several weeks as the child makes the transition to his new no-nap routine. Anticipate some evening temper tantrums brought on by fatigue—and hang onto your patience.

❋ TWO

*Bedtime Battles: How to
Make Sure You Both
Come Out Ahead*

If you are a parent whose child is difficult to get to sleep, you've probably experienced one of these scenarios:

- You nurse your baby to sleep and then, holding your breath, lay her gently in the crib. But the moment her head touches the mattress, she starts to scream.
- As you tuck your toddler under the covers, he clings to your arm and tearfully begs, "Stay, Daddy."
- You've already read more bedtime stories than you'd planned to, yet still your preschooler complains, "Is that all? I'm not going to bed until I hear all of *Aladdin*."

There are myriad reasons why children mutiny at bedtime. Fortunately, there are also a variety of ways to resolve such conflicts before full-scale battle erupts.

What if a state of war already exists in your household? The methods presented in this chapter can help you negotiate a peace treaty.

INFANTS ONLY: HELPING YOUR NEWBORN SETTLE DOWN FOR SLEEP

Through the nursery door you can hear her wails. You placed your infant in the crib a few minutes ago, and clearly she's not happy to be there. What do you do? First, check to see if she's in any discomfort.

Newborns are not very good at conserving body heat and may become chilled quickly. If you suspect she's having trouble falling asleep because she's uncomfortably cold, wrap her in an extra blanket and raise the heat in her room slightly. If she tends to kick off her covers and then become chilled, put her to bed in pajamas with feet and long sleeves. Does she startle or cry out when first laid on her mattress? Try warming the sheet slightly with a heating pad, or cover the sheet with a receiving blanket you've just taken out of the clothes dryer.

But take care not to overdress your newborn, either; being overheated also makes it hard to sleep. Test this by touching the back of the baby's neck. If it is damp, he's probably too warm. A good rule of thumb: dress a baby in as many layers as you would find comfortable in the same setting, plus one extra layer such as a receiving blanket.

Now check the diaper. A slight amount of wetness shouldn't interfere with sleep, but do change a diaper that is very wet or at all soiled. Painful diaper rash can prevent peaceful settling, so if your baby's bottom is prone to this, apply protective ointment generously. Cloth diaper users, make sure the pin is not poking her or the Velcro closure scratching her. For disposable diapers, check to see if the sticky tab is stuck to her skin, if the corner of the tab is poking her tummy, or if its edge is digging into her thigh.

A stomach full of gas can keep an uncomfortable infant awake. This may have been an infrequent occurrence in previous years when babies were routinely put to bed on their tummies, because the pressure of the mattress against the abdomen often releases the gas. But now that doctors are recommending that infants sleep on their backs (see Chapter Five for more information), the problem of air bubbles interfering with sleep is perhaps more common.

To avoid this, try burping the cranky baby to see if this helps her settle down. If gas seems to be a chronic problem, burp your baby more frequently during feedings, and again at the end. Experiment with various positions—upright against your shoulder, face down across your lap, seated on your lap with one of your hands against her tummy—until you find the one that seems most effective at releasing your baby's air bubble.

Investigate other possible pains as well. Is his hand or foot caught between the mattress and crib slats? Crib bumpers can prevent this. Has he outgrown his sleeper, so that the neck and crotch areas are irritatingly tight? Is the fabric scratchy, or does a button or pompom press on some tender spot when he's lying down? Also check to see if the baby has a string or hair wrapped around a finger, toe, or his penis. This can cut off circulation, a painful and potentially dangerous situation that will certainly prevent the baby from falling asleep.

Or it may be that the baby is simply too wound up to settle down. Try rocking her or singing to her. Snuggle her with her head nestled in your neck and your chin resting over her head, and hum softly. Or drape her over your chest and place her ear over your heart; the combination of the rhythmic heartbeat and the movement of your chest as you breathe may help her settle down enough to sleep.

But don't carry such soothing too far. Your goal is not to have her fall asleep in your arms, but rather to calm her down to the point that she can go quietly into her crib and fall asleep there. The importance of this distinction will become clear later in this chapter, when the concept of sleep associations is discussed.

TALES OF BEDTIME RESISTANCE

If you are the parent of a once-great sleeper, know that a change in going-to-sleep patterns is not unusual. That's what Julia Martin, a mother of two, discovered. "Tess had always been our bedtime angel—sleeping through the night at 6 weeks, napping long and well during the day, going to bed each evening without a fuss. Then when she was 2½, it all fell apart," recalls Julia. "All of a sudden we were going through 12 different versions of 'Mommy, don't leave yet.' She'd say, 'I need a glass of water. Now I need to go potty. Close my curtains. No, don't close them that much. I don't have my bunny; let's go downstairs and look for it. Daddy didn't kiss me good night yet. That kiss didn't count, so I need another.' She was driving my husband and me crazy."

AGE FLAG: 18 TO 36 MONTHS

Tess isn't the only formerly compliant tot to suddenly begin resisting bedtime. Around age 2, a toddler begins his struggle for independence from his parents, and often that struggle includes a refusal to do anything Mom or Dad wants him to do, such as go quietly to bed. He's also become more savvy; he has realized that, through his protests, he can postpone bedtime and receive extra attention from his parents.

AGE FLAG: 3 TO 5 YEARS

Moving ahead to the preschool years, a child may be further motivated to resist bedtime because he doesn't want to "miss out on the action." "By this age, the child becomes more acutely aware of the fact that he is alone upstairs while his parents are together downstairs. And he'll probably protest this isolation all the more if older siblings are still awake when his parents are putting him to bed," says Dr. Amy Wolfson. At this age, stalling is quite common—a *Child* magazine survey reports that more than 50 percent of preschoolers engage in such tactics—and the ruses used become more contrived and elaborate.

These manipulations may leave you bewildered about what to do, so you wind up being wishy-washy one night and adamant the next. Yet such inconsistency only proves to the child that her will to resist can at times outlast your energy for enforcing the rules. So she badgers you even more, hoping tonight will be one of those times.

Bedtime represents a particularly difficult adjustment for any child whose parents are less than effective at setting limits during the day. "In the course of the day, it often may seem to a parent that capitulating to the child's wishes is the easiest way to avoid conflict. But then at night, when this parent tries to impose more definitive limits, the child rebels because he's not used to following rules," explains Dr. John Herman. "From the child's perspective, it appears that he has been controlling things all day—then suddenly at night, his parents stage a guerrilla uprising to seize control of the household and exile him to a dark and dreary solitary confinement."

Even parents who have no trouble setting limits during the day may be so eager for the youngster to sleep at night that they give in to anything—not realizing they're really reinforcing the child's rebellious behavior. Single mother Thalia Davis (not her real name) admits, "My 2½-year-old son is basically an agreeable, cooperative child, but he won't comply with any kind of bedtime rules. He refuses to go to sleep when I tell him to, and throws terrible tantrums if I try to make him stay in his room. So now I let him stay up until I'm tired, then I put him in bed with me. Usually I fall asleep around 11 P.M., but often he stays awake. Sometimes I wake up long after midnight and find him still playing next to me in the bed. I know this is a bad situation, but I've given up. I just don't have the strength to fight it."

Giving up is no solution, but fortunately you do have other options. One of the most simple, pleasant, and effective of these is the establishment of a regular bed-time routine or ritual.

WHY THE BEDTIME ROUTINE IS INDISPENSABLE

"The bedtime ritual helps children learn to be sleepy at bedtime," explains Dr. Jodi Mindell. "Human circadian rhythms actually operate on a 25-hour day. To help ourselves click back to a 24-hour schedule, adults watch the clock. But young kids can't tell time. For them, a nightly ritual signals that it's time to wind down."

To a child, sleep represents a kind of deprivation—the loss of her parents' company, the loss of playtime. The bedtime ritual helps offset her sense of loss by providing her with something she craves: a half-hour of undivided attention from Mom and Dad. By ending her day on a happy note and associating bedtime with positive experiences, she can drift toward sleep secure in the knowledge of her family's love.

AGE FLAG: 3 TO 6 MONTHS AND UP

Although rebellion is not a cause of bedtime crying in infants—they're too young to employ such manipulative tactics—it's wise to begin a nightly routine early on. "As a young infant, your child may fall asleep anywhere and any time he's tired, but this won't last forever. If you establish a settling-down routine when the baby is 3 to 6 months old, it will be in place by the time you really need it," says Dr. Mindell.

The specifics of what is included in the routine are less important than its consistency. A child may become downright rigid about his going-to-sleep ritual; if you vary it on any given evening, he may get upset or even have trouble going to sleep. Audrey Cope, a mother of one, confesses, "If I'm in a good mood, I may read five or six books to my son at bedtime. But if I'm tired or eager to have some private time with my husband, I resent it when William insists on more than one or two books." Your best bet: select activities you're willing to repeat night after night after night, and stick with them.

It's also important to leave enough time in your evening schedule for the entire ritual. If you want to establish a bedtime of 8:30, for instance, you'll have to start the ritual well before that time. Be advised: few parents can get away with a super-quickie ritual, as my sister Barbara learned. "As I planned my evening, I used to allot 10 minutes to put Peter to bed. Of course he would do everything possible to drag it out, and I wouldn't get back downstairs for an hour. Each nightly struggle ended with my feeling aggravated and my son feeling rejected," says Barbara. "Finally I decided to devote 30 minutes to his bedtime routine, and now we both enjoy the whole process more. I don't feel annoyed about 'wasting' time, and he's thrilled with this half-hour of undivided attention. Best of all, he goes to bed with far fewer protests than before."

Understand that your participation in the ritual is essential. "Yelling over the top of your newspaper 'Go on, brush your teeth and go to bed' will never work as well as putting down the paper and walking your child into the bathroom and then into the bedroom," notes Dr. Charles E. Schaefer. Not only are you more likely to be obeyed, but your child is able to end her day with a warm sense of being loved and cared for.

Better yet, have both parents participate actively in the routine. Otherwise, the time will come when the more involved parent is out for the evening, and the child will have a very hard time settling down to sleep for the other parent. My sister Barbara learned this lesson from her 2-year-old daughter: "I made a big mistake in not getting my husband involved in Caroline's bedtime routine from the beginning. The first time Dick tried to put her to bed, she was so unnerved by this unfamiliar experience that she took off her diaper, poohed in her crib, then smeared it all over the wall." If your child feels that only Mommy or only Daddy will do, try gradually involving the other parent by having him take over first one and then another of the scheduled bedtime activities, until the child accepts either parent doing the whole routine.

At what point will your child outgrow her bedtime routine? Probably not for many years. "We've had essentially the same ritual for our daughter since she was 6 months old—bath, book, prayer, and song—and now she's 9 years old," says Dr. May Griebel. Obviously, a school-age child may ask you to read *Little Women* instead of *The Little Engine That Could*, but the basic format of the routine remains unchanged.

How to Structure a Bedtime Routine

The bedtime routine begins long before the toothbrushing and storybook-reading; it begins with the build-up. And that build-up should be a quiet one. "Reserve the hour before bedtime for quiet play. This lowers your child's activity level and prepares his nervous system for relaxation. Roughhousing, running, and tickling games make a peaceful transition to sleep especially difficult," explains Dr. Schaefer. After dinner, encourage your child to look at books, play quiet board games, do puzzles, listen to music. If watching TV is allowed, be sure the show is not overly stimulating. Don't let the child begin any lengthy project that he'll have trouble leaving unfinished.

Next, get the necessities out of the way. A child will be more motivated to cooperate with the hygiene routine if he knows the fun stuff will follow. "If your child is accustomed to taking a bath in the evening and finds this soothing, fine. But if he hates to bathe or is very stimulated by it, reschedule the bath for earlier in the day," suggests Dr. Mindell. After the teeth are brushed (or for an infant, the gums wiped with a clean, damp cloth) and the diaper changed or potty used, it's P.J. time. Allowing the child to select which pajamas to wear gives him a sense of control and makes the whole process more enjoyable for him. Of course, praise him for cooperating with all these preparations.

Perform the rest of the ritual in the child's own bedroom. "If you do the most enjoyable parts of the routine in another room and then pop the child into bed, his room becomes a cage, a place to which he is banished when the fun is over. But if you use his room as the scene for the fun, he will associate his room with happy, comforting times. And that will make it easier for him to fall asleep there," says Dr. Mindell.

Your ritual might include reading books, reciting poems, singing songs. Even an infant too young to understand the words will be soothed by the rhythms and the sound of your voice. Toddlers may like to hear the same favorite story night after night while preschoolers often opt for new tales. Keep in mind that as tempting as watching TV together may be, especially if you're tired, it is a very poor substitute for interactive activities like reading or singing.

Next, you might offer your child a last drink of water, suggest another visit to the potty, and ask if there's anything else she needs. Then tuck her into bed with lots of hugs and kisses. Use these final few minutes to sing a last lullaby to an infant, or to encourage close conversation with an older child. "By the time a child is 2, she can talk with you about what she did that day and what she'll be doing tomorrow," notes Dr. Mindell. You could suggest to the child three good things to think about as she falls asleep, tell her three things about herself that you find wonderful, or have her name all the people who love her. Then kiss her one last time.

If you have several children, each with his own bedtime, you might opt to do a short individual routine with each child. When youngsters are close in age and share a bedtime, as in my family, it may work best to do one big ritual all together, then finish with some one-on-one snuggling and talking during the tucking-in.

AGE FLAG: 3 MONTHS TO 3 YEARS

A ritual is useful at naptime, too, because it helps the child calm down and signals to him that it is time for sleep. You needn't go through your entire bedtime routine before each nap, but do follow some sort of standard procedure—for instance, reading one story, tucking the child in, and giving him a good-nap kiss.

A Typical Countdown-to-Bedtime Routine

7:15—Quiet play
7:45—Wash up
7:55—Put on pajamas
8:00—Brush teeth
8:05—Read books in child's room
8:20—Final trip to potty; last drink of water
8:25—Tuck in: lullaby, prayers, or ritual naming of loved ones
8:30—Last kiss, lights out

Avoiding the "Just One More" Syndrome

If your child asks for a change in the ritual, incorporate his requests if at all possible. But beware of escalation, a process through which the ritual gradually grows beyond your established bounds. It's easy to spot by the "just one more" requests for a story, a drink, a potty break.

"Recently, I counseled the parents of a 2-year-old on the importance of establishing a bedtime ritual. When they came back to see me the following week, they admitted their child had stretched the routine to include 3 hours of reading each night," says Dr. Mindell. Naturally, you'll need to set limits on the bedtime ritual, just as you must on daytime behavior. For example, tell the child in advance that you'll read one story and sing one song, and then it's lights out.

"I learned that it helps to phrase these limits in a positive way," adds my sister Barbara. "Now I say, 'Oh, how lucky, we have time to read this whole book tonight!' instead of, 'I'm only going to read you this one little book and that's it.'"

For some families, a father or mother's late-evening arrival can interrupt the bedtime routine, making it drag out longer than it normally would. Jennifer Trillo, a mother of three preschool girls, explains, "I'm never sure what time my husband will get home from work at night. If he arrives before I start getting the girls ready for bed, they all play together for a while, and that's fine. Or if he shows up after they're asleep, there's no problem. The trouble occurs on the nights he drives up just as I'm finishing the bedtime routine. I'll have the kids all calmed down and ready for bed, but when they hear that garage door open—boom! It's like somebody shot them out of a cannon. They're so excited to see their dad that they don't settle down again until I go through the entire ritual a second time."

If you share this problem, a bit of scheduling coordination can help. Ask your partner to phone home with an estimated time of arrival each evening. Then you can push bedtime forward a bit so the kids are asleep before your partner arrives, or you can plan to delay bedtime a little so the children can play with the other parent briefly before bed. Either way, you'll have to go through the ritual only once.

Your child still finds endless ways to stretch the bed-time routine each night? Honestly evaluate the amount of time you spend with her during the day, suggests Dr. Deborah Madansky. "If the only time she gets your attention is at bedtime, naturally she'll go to great lengths to try to prolong the routine." If you can find an extra 15 minutes to focus on her during the day, you lessen her need to escalate the bedtime activities.

Should a Child's Bedroom Be Used as a Place for Punishment?

Today's parents are likely to impose a bedroom-based time-out. But as disciplinary tactics go, sending a child to his room may be counterproductive. Why? Because it can lead to sleep problems. "A bedroom that's used as a place for punishment becomes a jail. The child associates his room with feelings of anger and rejection during the day—feelings that make it impossible for him to feel secure and content in bed at night," explains Dr. Martin Scharf. Better bet: choose a less emotionally charged location for time-outs, such as a corner in the kitchen, a chair in the hallway, or the bottom step of the staircase.

SLEEP ASSOCIATIONS: HOW THEY AFFECT A CHILD'S ABILITY TO FALL ASLEEP

When I get ready for bed each night, I make sure everything is just the way it's supposed to be: front door locked, bathroom door open, night light on, hall light off. I lie on the left side of the bed, fluff my pillow, check the clock, read for a while, then kiss my husband good night, and turn out the bedside lamp. Usually, sleep comes quickly. But on those nights when something's not as it should be—the night light's burned out, or my husband's away, or the new sheets feel unfamiliar—falling asleep takes longer.

Everyone has such sleep associations, or conditions under which they are accustomed to falling asleep. For some people, a change in bedtime conditions is no big deal, but for others, such a change makes falling asleep almost impossible.

Sleep associations often are established early in life, as parents discover that their child falls asleep more readily under certain circumstances—for instance, when she's being rocked or nursed or sung to. Because the parents are probably eager for the baby to sleep, they willingly provide that rocking, that breast, that song. The problem is, if your child's sleep associations involve your active participation, she will be unable to fall asleep without your help. By "putting" your child to sleep, you rob her of her innate ability to fall asleep by herself. This means that, every time you want to put her down, you have to re-create the conditions she's accustomed to. What's worse, every time she wakes in the middle of the night, she'll cry for you to re-establish those same conditions, because without them, she cannot go back to sleep. (See Chapter Three for more on how sleep associations affect nighttime wakings.)

"My husband, Michael, created a monster," Ann Stirling says with a sigh. "He got into the habit of scratching our son's back every night until the baby dozed off. It got to the point where Ian couldn't fall asleep any other way. Michael or I had to sit by his bed scratching, scratching, scratching, sometimes for 20 minutes or longer. If we tried to tiptoe away too soon, before Ian was fully asleep, the little guy would cry and we'd have to start all over again. If we refused, he'd scream and scream until we gave in. Ian was absolutely addicted."

Obviously, this type of dependency represents a huge inconvenience for parents. Sandy Dotson, a mother of two, says, "I've always sung to my daughters at bedtime, from the time they were newborn babies. Our limit is five lullabies, and the idea is for them to fall asleep before the fifth song is over. But sometimes they don't fall asleep that fast, so I have to keep singing and singing and singing. Many a night, I sit there in an agony of frustration, feeling trapped and thinking of all the dozens of other things I need to get done that evening."

Sounds familiar? Unfortunately, if you're hoping you can simply grit your teeth and stick it out until your child outgrows his dependency, you're probably in for a long, long wait. Ann Stirling's son didn't break the back-scratching habit until he was 6 years old; Sandy Dotson's two daughters, now 5 and 3, are still falling asleep to the sound of their mom's voice.

AGE FLAG: 5 YEARS AND UP

Some parents of older kids, in an attempt to free themselves of this time-consuming nightly commitment, establish a new policy that allows the children to watch TV until sleep comes. "Judging by the large numbers of children who fall asleep at the tube, this is a seemingly effective and easy solution. But in fact it creates more problems than it remedies," says Dr. Schaefer.

For one thing, if the program is interesting enough, the child will stay awake far too late. What's more, there will certainly be situations in which the child cannot watch TV until he passes out, such as when he spends the night at a friend's house or attends sleep-away camp. And the fact remains that the child still has not learned how to get to sleep on his own.

Strategies for Getting a Child to Fall Asleep on Her Own

Fortunately, this is a skill that can be taught. And the younger your child is when you begin to teach her, the more easily the lesson will be learned. Here are two important steps to take:

1. Put the child to bed drowsy but not asleep.

   AGE FLAG: NEWBORN TO 1 YEAR

   With an infant, this can be a tough assignment, because he's likely to fall asleep while you feed him. Keep him awake if possible. If he seems determined to doze, end the feeding and lay him down while he's still somewhat aware. You want him to know that he is in his crib, not in your arms; you want his last waking memory to be of his bedroom and blankets, not of your breast or a bottle.

AGE FLAG: 1 YEAR AND UP

With an older child, the goal is the same: to let him be aware of the fact that, as he falls asleep, he is snug and secure in his own bed—and that you are not there in the room with him. What if he wants you to stay? "It's fine to linger a little while, provided you set a limit—for example, by telling the child you'll sit with him for 5 minutes," says Dr. Ferber. "But if you say you'll stay until he falls asleep, he may fight drowsiness in order to keep you with him longer. And he still won't figure out how to fall asleep on his own."

Admittedly, this advice sounds absurd to parents desperate to get a fussy child to sleep. If you're completely wiped out by evening and your child doesn't seem to be adjusting easily to the change in his bedtime routine, begin this phase of sleep training during the day. Continue your usual putting-the-child-to-sleep tricks in the evening for now, but during the day, put him down for his naps while he's drowsy. Once he's used to falling asleep on his own in the daytime, the new nighttime policy should be less troublesome to implement.

2. Encourage the use of a soother that doesn't require your presence. Cultivate a relationship between your child and some special object such as a toy or blanket. Once she has bonded with a "lovey," it becomes a symbolic replacement for her parents and enables her to soothe herself when she's alone in her room at bedtime. What's more, she'll appreci-

ate the fact that Teddy doesn't get up and walk away after she's asleep, the way a parent does.

Embarrassed to see your child drag around that tattered blanket or grungy teddy bear? Don't be. "Some parents worry that the need for a lovey is a sign of an insecure personality, yet studies show that this is not true," says Dr. Schaefer. "In fact, as she struggles to leave your protective arms and find ways to calm her own fears, a security object is an 'emotionally mature' way to leap toward independence."

You can offer your child several types of security objects, but you must let him choose for himself which is to be the favorite. As an infant, my daughter Samantha was indifferent to the teddy in a tutu I brought home from a fancy toy store, and to the rainbow-hued blanket her grandmother had lovingly crocheted. Instead, what caught her fancy was a blue pug-nose pig someone (I can't even remember who) had given to her twin brother. Piggy is now a faded blue-gray, and his stuffing is forever falling out—but Samantha loves him and sleeps with him still.

Experts often advise that, whenever possible, parents procure a second lovey identical to the one their child adores. I learned my lesson after several anxious bedtime searches for a misplaced Piggy. So when my son, James, fell in love with a blue die-cast train engine, I bought several extras to use in emergencies.

* * *

Here are a variety of self-soothers in which your child might take comfort:

- *Pacifier.* Many babies seem to have a need to suck that is not completely satisfied during feedings, and for them a pacifier can be quite calming. But beware: when the pacifier gets lost under the blankets or falls out of the crib, the baby may cry for you to come in and retrieve it—precisely the opposite of the self-soothing behavior you're trying to promote. To prevent such problems, use a pacifier clip; one end snaps around the ring of the pacifier, and the other end clips onto the baby's pajamas. (Never use any string longer than 12 inches, to avoid the risk of strangulation.) Or you might place several pacifiers in the crib at bedtime, upping the odds that your baby will be able to find at least one without help. Some brands glow in the dark, making them easier to locate in an unlit bedroom. Check the pacifiers every day for signs of weakening, since a worn pacifier could break apart and present a choking hazard.
- *Thumb.* The advantage to thumb-sucking is that the thumb never wears out or gets lost. The disadvantage is that, if the child does not outgrow the habit by the time he starts school, it may cause him much embarrassment and angst, as well as potential orthodontic problems.
- *Blanket.* This universal favorite might be as fancy as the beautiful quilt my mother made for my youngest son Jack, or as simple as the receiving blanket you wrapped your newborn babe in at the hospital. Some babies even prefer the shoulder cloth you used to burp her after a feeding, if it's not messy, since it

contains your scent as well as her own. *(Note: do not offer a pillow to any child under the age of 2, since it poses a suffocation risk.)*

- *Stuffed animal.* Some youngsters love the traditional teddy; others prefer more exotic furry friends. To avoid the risk of choking, be sure all buttons are very securely attached and that there are no small parts that might be pulled off.
- *Sound.* Constant soft sound—a white-noise machine, the hum of a fan—can be soothing to some babies. Others enjoy the noise of a vacuum cleaner or car engine; make a tape recording so you don't have to sweep the rugs or go for a drive every time you want your baby to sleep. My neighbor, Venice Phillips, installed a lighted fish tank in her son Ryan's room, and let the gurgling bubbles lull him to sleep. But take note: do not let your child come to rely on any sound-maker you're unwilling to leave on all night or on a music box that you have to rewind.
- *Rhythmic movement.* Studies reveal that as many as two-thirds of 9-month-old babies regularly show some type of rhythmic body movement—head rolling, body rocking, hair stroking, head banging—as they settle into sleep or transition from one sleep cycle to the next. Most children outgrow these behaviors by age 4, and in general parents have no cause for concern. The one exception is head banging. "Injuries among head bangers are uncommon, but if a child is hurting himself this way, a soft helmet and crib pads can help," says Dr. Griebel.

When Your Child Refuses to Go to Sleep Without You

You've made sure your child is comfortable, you've established an attentive bedtime ritual, you've encouraged her to bond with her chosen security object—yet still she cries and complains unless you do whatever it is she is accustomed to having you do in order to put her to sleep. What next?

The experts' opinions vary widely, and some, in fact, are diametrically opposed. So you need to make a decision—and it's a very personal decision. What worked for your sister might not work for you. What's recommended by your pediatrician might just feel wrong to you.

First consider your own overall approach to child rearing. Are you a no-nonsense type who likes to confront problems head on? Or a tenderhearted nurturer who hates to hear a baby cry? Next, consider the pros and cons of the methods outlined below. What are the practical aspects involved in each? What is the parents' role in making the method succeed? Now choose the method that feels right to you. Promise yourself that you'll stick with it for 2 weeks; the problem will probably be solved or at least noticeably improved within that time. If it isn't, choose another method and start again.

THE CRY-IT-OUT METHOD

AGE FLAG: 6 MONTHS TO 2½ YEARS

Some parents select this method right from the start. Some refuse to do this under any circumstances. Others may try it only if they aren't successful with alternative techniques. I describe the cry-it-out method first not because I favor its use over all others, but because it is the simplest to understand and to implement, requiring almost no active participation on the parents' part. It's most effective for children who sleep in a crib and cannot yet climb out.

Here's what you do: put the baby to bed at a reasonable hour, say good night affectionately but firmly, walk out of the room, and don't go back. Yes, the child will cry. No, you should not go back in to comfort her, feed her, hold her, or talk to her. You let her cry until she falls asleep on her own, no matter whether that takes 2 minutes or 2 hours.

The cry-it-out method is based on two beliefs: that unwanted behavior that is ignored will die out; and that a reasonable amount of crying does not hurt a child. If you subscribe to this philosophy, this method may be appropriate for you.

First, select a convenient time to implement the new policy. Choose a time when the child is healthy, and when there has been no recent upheaval such as a move to a new home or the start of daycare. If you live in an apartment or town house, you may want to explain your plans to your neighbors, so they won't be unduly concerned when they hear the baby's wailing. Be sure the child has her security object with her in the crib, because now is when she needs it most.

The cry-it-out method is usually quite effective and relatively quick. The baby may scream for several hours the first night or two, but often by the third or fourth night the crying is much reduced. Dr. Wolfson notes, "Many parents resist this approach because it sounds so drastic. They envision their child sobbing all night for the next hundred nights. In truth, the child learns very quickly, usually within a few nights." By that point, a child will probably go to bed with a minimum of fussing—having learned that he can indeed fall asleep without being rocked or nursed or sung or back-scratched into oblivion.

What effect does prolonged crying have on the child? Again, expert opinion is divided and no one knows for sure. But proponents of the method argue that, when parents are appropriately nurturing during the day, it causes the child no psychological or physical harm for his parents to ignore his nighttime protests.

In fact, the method may be hardest on the parents. "The first night my 9-month-old son cried for an hour and a half. I sat in my room with my fists clenched, and my teeth clenched, aching to pick him up. But I knew I shouldn't. I had to put a stop to the nightly craziness we'd been living with up till then," says Cathy Gardner (not her real name), a mother of two.

To survive the first grueling night or two, try following these tips:

• Time your baby's crying. Many parents are surprised to realize that what seemed to them to be several hours of screaming was in fact just 45 minutes.
• Use a white-noise machine, radio, or TV to cover up the sound of the cries. Or wear earplugs, removing them periodically to find out if the crying has stopped. If you normally use a baby monitor, turn it off. Every 15 minutes, switch it back on briefly to see whether the baby has fallen asleep yet.

- Most parents can readily distinguish between a cry of pain and a cry of anger or frustration. You can safely let the angry screams go unanswered. But if the cry changes to one of pain, check on the child immediately to make sure she's all right.
- Remember, as discussed in Chapter One, young children can go from bellowing wakefulness to sound sleep much faster than an adult can. Console yourself with the knowledge that those bloodcurdling howls may die down suddenly at any moment, as the child falls asleep.

There are instances in which the cry-it-out method should not be attempted:

- When the baby is less than 6 months old.
- When you have a spouse or nearby neighbor who insists on not being disturbed.
- When you are ambivalent about the method and unsure of your ability to stick with it. "It's not helpful to let the baby scream for an hour and then, overcome with guilt, rush in to pick him up and apologize for upsetting him so," notes Dr. Madansky. "This only teaches the child that if he screams long enough, he'll eventually get what he wants."

THE REASSURING APPROACH

AGE FLAG: 6 MONTHS TO 2½ YEARS

Many parents feel the cry-it-out method is too harsh—and many experts agree. "I'm not comfortable with cold-turkey tactics. It's too drastic to go from one extreme of being fully available to your baby whenever he cries for you to the other extreme of not being available at all for 10 hours," explains Dr. Ferber. While the child does learn to fall asleep without help, some experts fear that he does so at the expense of his sense of security and trust in his parents.

The reassuring approach, on the other hand, is intended to convey a gentler message: "There is no need to cry. We have not deserted you. We will always come back, though we won't always come immediately. But now it's time for you to go to sleep in your crib."

How does this message get through? The parents do not take the child out of the crib, nor do they actively participate in putting the child to sleep. Instead, they visit the nursery at regular intervals to reassure their child of their presence and their love. The child may feel unhappy at the change in his nightly routine, and he may well cry for some time, but he will not feel abandoned or frightened.

This method is appropriate for children over the age of 6 months who still sleep in a crib. (At the end of this chapter we discuss variations appropriate for older children.) It is not recommended for a youngster who's afraid of the dark or who has separation anxiety. (See Chapter Four for tips on handling these problems.)

Choose a convenient time to begin—not when you have weekend visitors or an important meeting at work the next day. Forewarn any neighbors within earshot, so they won't be alarmed to hear the crying. Be sure you and your spouse agree on the approach and are both willing to work at it.

The most popular version of this approach is the one devised by Dr. Ferber. In fact, satisfied parents have elevated his name to a verb: "We've Ferberized our baby, and now we're all sleeping better." Here's what you do:

Step 1. Put the child to bed in his crib when he's drowsy but not yet asleep. Say good night and leave the room. If he cries (which he almost certainly will if he's accustomed to falling asleep with your help), wait 5 minutes and then return to the nursery.

Step 2. Speaking calmly and very quietly, reassure the child that he is all right and that you are near. Direct his attention to his lovey, and then remind him it is time to sleep. Do not turn on any lights (other than a night light), and do not take the child out of the crib. Leave the room after no more than 1 or 2 minutes, even if the child is still crying. Do not stay with him until he falls asleep. The goal is for him to fall asleep when you are not in the room.

Step 3. If the crying continues, wait 10 more minutes. When the time is up, go back into the nursery and repeat the brief verbal comforting process, again without picking up the baby. Then leave the room once more.

Step 4. If he still hasn't stopped crying, wait 15 minutes. Return to his room to reassure him, then leave again. Continue comforting him at 15-minute intervals until he falls asleep during one of the waiting periods during which you are not in his room. (If the crying fades to a whimper, do not go back into the nursery unless he starts to wail once more.)

Step 5. On the second night, let the child cry for 10 minutes before going to his room to reassure him for the first time. If he continues to fuss, stretch the next interval to 15 minutes, and the third and all subsequent intervals to 20 minutes.

Step 6. On the third night, wait for 15 minutes before entering his room to comfort him the first time. Lengthen the second interval to 20 minutes, and the third and all subsequent intervals to 25 or 30 minutes.

What can you expect when using the reassuring approach? The first night or two can be stressful, since the child may cry for an hour or more. Yet by the third night, she may well be going to sleep much sooner— and with far less fussing. "I used this method when my son was 6 months old, and it worked like a textbook case. After three nights, Cole was going to bed with no crying, and we haven't had any problems since," says Beth Ava, mother of one.

Other parents may find that progress comes more slowly, particularly if there are numerous sleep associations that need to be corrected. A child who is used to having a parent hold her hand until she falls asleep, for example, may learn more quickly than a child who's dependent on being nursed, stroked, and sung to simultaneously.

Beth Turchi, mother of one daughter, shares her experience: "Each night, I had to feed Lilly until she was drowsy, then give her a pacifier and rock her until she fell asleep. This went on for 8 months. Once I finally decided to break her of the rocking habit, I figured I might as well tackle the bottle habit and pacifier habit at the same time. After all, I knew she'd cry about not being rocked—so why not let her cry about all three things at once? It seemed more sensible to get it over with, instead of stringing things out by breaking each habit one at a time. It took 2 solid weeks, but by the end of that time, she no longer was crying at all when I put her to bed."

Guilt-stricken at the thought that your child might suffer psychological harm from the experience? That's highly unlikely. "This approach is not unkind or extreme. Crying is kept to a minimum because the child understands that you will return eventually," says Dr. Ferber. Remind yourself that this is one of those times when you as a parent must decide what's best for your child, even if he objects. "If a child is poking a nail into an electrical outlet, you're going to stop him, and you won't feel guilty about it no matter how much he cries. It's the same situation when you help a child learn to fall asleep on a mattress instead of in your arms. Though he complains at first, in the long run he'll be happier with more restful, pleasant nights."

Variations on the Theme— for Babies Not Yet Verbal

AGE FLAG: 6 TO 18 MONTHS

One of the beauties of the reassuring approach is that it can be modified in a variety of ways to suit your individual parenting style. Here are some suggestions:

- The 5/10/15-minute progressive schedule is not engraved in stone. If 5 minutes is longer than you can

comfortably listen to your baby howl, you can start
by letting your child cry for just 1 minute before
visiting her for the first time. Then wait 2 minutes,
then 3, then 4, and work your way up from there.
The important thing is for the schedule to be one that
both parents feel comfortable with and are willing to
stick to. It may take longer for your child to learn to
settle herself this way, but eventually success will
come.

- On the other hand, if you find all that clock-watching
and careful timing an annoyance, you needn't be so
precise about building up the waiting periods. "It's
simpler and just as effective to visit the child every
10 minutes or so, comfort her briefly, and then
leave," notes Dr. Madansky.

- Some experts recommend that you offer only verbal
reassurances during the periodic visits to the nursery—no back patting, no stroking, and certainly no
picking up—in order to avoid rewarding the child's
wakefulness with such positive attention. Many parents, however, find that they themselves feel more
reassured after they give the child a kiss on the head
or a pat on the back.

Cathy Gardner explains, "I had been advised not
to enter the nursery, but simply to whisper my words
of comfort while standing in the doorway. So I did.
But my 9-month-old son's crying went on and on and
on for hours that first night. Finally, I couldn't stand
it anymore. I went into his room and as soon as I
touched him, I realized he was burning up with fever.
I felt so terrible! Of course, that was the end of sleep
training for a while, until my son was completely
recovered from his illness. Finally, I felt ready to try

the method again—but I made certain that each time I visited his room, I gave him a hug or a kiss. That way I could be sure he wasn't running a temperature."

- What if you feel ready to try the reassuring approach to sleep training, but your spouse is too tenderhearted to follow through? Terry Capriotti, a mother of one, offers this suggestion: "My husband couldn't stand to hear our son cry. So when I decided to Ferberize Tony at 14 months, I chose a long weekend during which my husband was out of town. The baby did scream for quite a while those three nights—but by the time my husband got home, Tony was going to sleep on his own with scarcely a peep."

Variations on the Theme—
for Youngsters Old Enough to Talk

AGE FLAG: 18 MONTHS AND UP

Toddlers and preschoolers often respond well to a variation on the reassuring approach known as "checking." Here's a sample script to illustrate the process:

PARENT: (Tucks child into bed.) Good night, sweetheart. See you in the morning.

CHILD: Mommy, don't leave yet! Stay with me and hold my hand until I fall asleep.

PARENT: Honey, I can't do that. Remember, we talked about how important it was for you to learn to go to sleep on your own, without my needing to hold your hand every night anymore.

CHILD: But I like to have you here with me.

PARENT: I know what we can do. I'll leave now, but I'll
         come back in 5 minutes and check on you, just
         to make sure you're fine and to kiss you good
         night one more time.

CHILD: What if you forget to come back?

PARENT: I promise I won't forget. I'll set the kitchen timer
         to remind myself.

CHILD: Well, okay.

The purpose of this checking is to reassure your youngster of your presence, affection, and trustworthiness. "By enhancing her sense of security, you enable her to settle down to sleep more easily," says Dr. Mindell. "Of course, once you've struck this bargain, it's crucial that you do check in at the promised time."

Remember Julia Martin, whose daughter Tess launched a major bedtime rebellion for the first time at the age of 2½? Julia finally hit on the solution, a variation of this checking technique: "One night when Tess was crying and carrying on about not wanting me to leave her room, I told her, 'Honey, if you need me, just call and I will come.' Like magic, the hysteria stopped. She did test me on it of course, and I did have to go check on her a time or two each evening. But once she saw that she could trust me to come when she called, she didn't abuse the system."

Unfortunately, some kids do abuse the system, calling out repeatedly and not waiting for the promised check-in time. In such a case, Dr. Schaefer recommends a tactic called tapering. "Tell your child, 'If you do not call out after I've said good night, I'll come back to your room to see how you're doing every 15 minutes. But if you do call out, the 15-minute wait starts all over again.'"

Finally, keep in mind that one important key to success with all the sleep-training techniques described in this chapter is for you to keep your cool. Naturally, there will be times when you feel frustrated, even furious, with your child, yet the more you can keep your reactions under control, the more you'll be able to follow through with your chosen methods—and the more your child will gain the sense of security he needs if he is to learn healthier sleep habits.

THREE

*Managing
Middle-of-the-Night
Awakenings*

They moaned and groaned, they rolled their eyes, they clenched their fists and clutched their heads in agony. An emergency room at a busy hospital? No, the scene was my preschoolers' mommy-and-me playgroup, and I had just introduced the topic of children's nighttime wakings. Nearly every parent present had a tale to tell, and few of the stories were happy ones.

If you, too, have trouble with a child who habitually wakes up at night, and wakes you up as well, this chapter can help. But first you need to understand one physiological fact about sleep. Night wakings are inevitable; everyone, no matter what their age, wakes briefly several times during the course of every night. Therefore, you cannot completely prevent your child's nighttime wakings—but you can prevent him from turning those natural, normal, momentary wakings into endless, exasperating, exhausting ordeals that rob the entire family of needed rest.

INFANTS ONLY: NEWBORNS' NIGHTTIME NEEDS

My mother-in-law, Gloria Garvey, claims that her daughter Judy slept through the night from the time she came home from the hospital. A miracle? Absolutely. But then, Gloria deserved some divine intervention, since Judy was her seventh child.

Most of the rest of us, however, must accept as inevitable the fact that a newborn baby will awaken at least once (and more likely twice or thrice) in the course of a night. This occurs in part because a newborn simply does not have the physiological maturity to sleep more than a few hours at a stretch. He cannot yet consolidate his slumber long enough to cycle several times between deep and light sleep without coming fully awake. Nor does a newborn have a developed sense of day versus night, to help her match her body cycles to those of the sun and moon. She may even reverse those cycles, snoozing much of the day away and then sparkling with energy when the stars come out.

AGE FLAG: NEWBORN TO 2 MONTHS

Of course, hunger also plays an important role in a baby's sleep/wake patterns. In the vast majority of cases, there's no escaping around-the-clock feedings for the first 2 months because a newborn's stomach holds only enough to satisfy him for 3 to 4 hours. That means he'll probably wake up and want to be fed twice each night.

AGE FLAG: 2 TO 4 MONTHS

During the next couple of months, a single nighttime feeding is usually enough. Your baby may even be sleeping for a 6-hour stretch each night at this point—an accomplishment known as "settling"—and if she is, count your blessings. Provided your pediatrician is satisfied with her weight gain, there's no reason to worry about missing that 2 A.M. feeding. By age 4 months, most infants have reached this important milestone. Formula-fed babies may do so a bit sooner than breast-fed ones, because formula digests more slowly than breast milk.

AGE FLAG: 6 MONTHS

Nearly all babies are physiologically ready to sleep through for about 10 hours by age 6 months or by the time they reach 12 pounds, and many do just that. Unfortunately, many don't. It's important for parents to understand that, when a healthy baby of 6 months or older wakes up at night and demands food or attention, he is doing so not out of physiological need, but out of habit. (More on this later in this chapter.)

While you cannot control a baby's developmental readiness to sleep through the night, there are ways you can encourage rather than interfere with her emerging readiness. "Start the day she comes home from the hospital, by helping her begin to differentiate between day and night," suggests Dr. Deborah Madansky. Here's how.

Show That Daytime Is Active Time

In order to consolidate his sleep into nighttime, an infant must also consolidate his wakefulness into daytime. You can encourage this:

- Play, sing, and talk with your baby to keep her amused and awake. If daytime boredom leads to constant siestas, she won't be able to sleep well at night.
- If the baby has napped for more than 3 consecutive hours, wake her up and play with her. This helps her learn to save her longest sleep period for nighttime. To wake her, try picking her up and patting her back, changing her diaper, tickling her toes.
- Keep the house well lit during the day. Even when the baby is napping, leave her window shades up and curtains open.
- Don't hush household noises during the baby's naps. You can vacuum, turn on the radio, leave the phone on the hook, let siblings play in the next room. Not only does this encourage shorter daytime naps (and hence longer nighttime sleep), but it also makes daily life far more pleasant for the rest of the family since the baby won't learn to require complete silence in order to sleep.
- Do your best to keep the baby awake in the early evening, to increase the likelihood that he'll sleep longer at night. An after-dinner bath or some active playtime with Dad may chase away the drowsies for another hour or so.

Show That Nighttime Is Quiet Time

Three-time mom Robin Hardin is the voice of experience on this: "When my first child, Amie, cried to be fed at 2 A.M., I'd take her downstairs and watch TV while she nursed. But then she'd be wide awake and ready to play, so we wouldn't get back to bed for 3 hours. It didn't matter much. I wasn't working and had no other kids to take care of, so Amie and I could both sleep in till 10 A.M.

"But after my second child was born, I realized that big sister Amie was going to continue waking up at 6 A.M. as she was now accustomed to do, and that I'd have to get up with her—even if baby Nikki and I had just gone back to bed at 5. I figured out pretty quickly that I needed to keep things quiet during the nighttime feedings, then put the baby straight back to bed when she finished nursing. This way we were both asleep again within half an hour."

Here's how to send your newborn the appropriate nighttime message:

- Pull down the window shades at night, and keep the house relatively quiet.
- When he wakes up hungry, feed him by the glow of a night light or other very dim lamp.
- During nighttime feedings, don't play with the baby, sing loudly, or talk in an animated tone. Speak in a whisper and sing very softly, if at all. Leave the television and radio off.
- Change his diaper only if it is very wet or soiled. "My youngest daughter Molly often wakes at 3 A.M., having wet her diaper so thoroughly that her pajamas

and sheets are soaked, too. By the time I've got everything cleaned up, Molly's wide awake and ready to play," says Jennifer Trillo, a mother of three. To prevent this, use two cloth diapers together for extra absorbency, or try an ultra-absorbent disposable diaper. You might also place a feminine napkin or diaper insert inside the diaper to absorb some of the excess moisture.

Exercise Some Influence Over Baby's Nighttime Feeding Schedule

AGE FLAG: NEWBORN AND UP

Influencing your baby's nighttime feeding schedule is a controversial approach. "Parents committed to feeding their baby on demand may resist the idea of imposing any control over when the baby eats," says Dr. Amy Wolfson. They may envision a ravenous infant screaming in frustration while they themselves anxiously watch the clock and wait impatiently for that arbitrarily appointed feeding hour to arrive. Yet the technique described below, often called the focal feeding method, does not force a hungry baby to wait for food—though it may mean you occasionally offer her food before she demands it.

You can use this method from the day your baby is born. Here's how to proceed:

- Schedule the baby's last feeding of the evening at your own bedtime—for instance, at 11:00 P.M. Be sure to select a time when you can be consistently available for this focal feeding.

- Try to keep the baby awake for the 2 hours preceding the focal feeding. If she does fall asleep, wake her up at 11:00.
- Now give the baby a complete feeding. If she dozes off while nursing or taking her bottle, awaken her by jiggling her gently in your arms, wiping her forehead with a damp cloth, unwrapping her blanket, or changing her diaper.
- Follow this routine consistently every evening.

Your purpose is twofold. First, by making sure the baby's tummy is full in the late evening, you decrease the likelihood that hunger will wake him in the middle of the night. Second, the focal feeding allows you to exert gentle control over your infant's emerging schedule. Dr. Schaefer explains, "Suppose your baby is physically able to stretch his sleep pattern to a full 8 hours. If you finish the final feeding of the evening at 8 P.M. and then put the baby to bed, his 8-hour stretch will end at 4 A.M.—at which time it certainly will not seem to you as if the baby has slept 'through the night.' But by giving the focal feeding at 11 P.M., you help your baby sleep through to 7 A.M. For most parents, this is a far easier schedule to live with."

Coping Strategies: Share Nighttime Feeding Duties with Your Partner (Even Nursing Mothers Can)

For most mothers, the worst part about around-the-clock feedings is never getting a nice long stretch of uninterrupted sleep. If you're bottle-feeding, you can solve that problem fairly easily by getting your partner to do his share. Try alternating nights on duty: you take care of all the baby's needs on even-numbered dates, so he can sleep undisturbed; let him answer any late-night summons on odd-numbered dates, so you can get some consolidated rest. If one partner's daytime work is simply too demanding to accommodate a 50-50 split in nighttime responsibilities, at least have that partner handle all the feedings on Friday and Saturday nights.

Some couples prefer to split the shift, as Lisa and Pat McDonough did. Lisa explains, "Nighttimes were especially exhausting because we had newborn twins, as well as two preschoolers. We were better able to cope when we divided the nighttime duties into two shifts. For instance, on weekends, Pat would take care of all the kids' needs from 9 P.M. to 2 A.M., while I slept. Then I'd manage everything from 2 A.M. to 7 A.M., while he slept."

A nursing mother can take advantage of such job-sharing arrangements by expressing milk and freezing it, or by supplementing with formula for the nighttime feedings. In fact, even if you're exclusively breast-feeding and your baby never takes a bottle, there's no need for you to shoulder the full burden. Your partner can get up when a hungry baby howls, bring her to you, burp her when she's finished eating, change her if she's wet, and settle her back into her crib. All you have to do on your "off-duty" nights is lie in bed next to your baby and doze while she nurses.

RETRAINING THE "TRAINED NIGHT FEEDER"

Earlier in this chapter, we explained that, by age 6 months, the vast majority of healthy babies are physiologically capable of sleeping through the night. However, a great many continue to wake up and demand food or attention—not because they truly need it, but because they have grown accustomed to having it. It's a sad fact that, by their first birthday, a full 10 percent of babies have not yet slept for 6 hours straight.

Do you have one of those babies? First, consider what it is your child cries for when he wakes at night. If he wants to be fed, you need to study this section on trained night feeders. If he wants to be comforted or played with, refer to the section in this chapter, Quieting the "Trained Night Crier" (page 91).

A trained night feeder is a child who, based on his age and size, no longer has any true physiological need to be fed around the clock but who nonetheless continues to cry for food in the middle of the night. He is simply accustomed to having food available 24 hours a day. As long as you are willing to serve as his all-night caterer, he'll keep coming back for more.

The trained night feeder phenomenon often gets its start when parents misinterpret "feed on demand" to mean "feed the baby every time she cries." The result: they pop a nipple in the baby's mouth in response to every squawk, rather than look for other ways to remedy his discontent. Soon the baby gets used to grazing—eating a small amount every hour or even every half-hour, rather than following the more typical pattern of having a full feeding every 3 to 4 hours. "Once this kind of snacking schedule is established, the baby will have trouble learning to fill his stomach in one feeding, preferring small continuous feedings," says Dr. Schaefer.

And the pattern can persist for many months. Just ask Suzanne Chester (not her real name), mother of one son: "At 7 months, Kevin was eating every 2 hours—at 6 A.M., 8 A.M., 10 A.M., noon, and so on through the afternoon and evening. At night, he did a little better—8 P.M., 11 P.M., 2 A.M. But still it seemed to me he should be able, at that age, to sleep all night without eating."

Grazers like Kevin aren't the only ones who become trained night feeders; picky eaters do, too. "As a baby, my younger daughter, Grace, didn't seem to eat as much or as often as my older daughter had done at the same age," says Marey Oakes, mother of four. "I figured she was waking at 2 A.M. to nurse because she wasn't getting enough to eat during the day. So even though she was almost a year old, I kept getting up every night to feed her."

What harm is there in having a trained night feeder in your home? If you've got one, you already know how draining it can be. It's hard enough for parents to survive those first few months with a newborn, when every night's sleep starts too late, ends too early, and is broken up too often. But when that disruption lasts for close to a year, or even longer, the physical and emotional stress level soars into the stratosphere.

Nor is this situation beneficial to the baby. "By age 6 months, a normal healthy baby should no longer need to consume great quantities of milk during the night," says Dr. Ferber. "To do so stimulates the digestive system at a time when it should be resting. This disrupts the body's normal rhythms and puts the baby in a state similar to chronic jet lag."

Before you tackle the problem, check with your pediatrician to verify that your baby is old enough, heavy enough, and growing rapidly enough to dispense with the nighttime feedings. If she's 4 months old and weighs more than 11½ pounds, you'll probably get the go-ahead; if she's over 6 months old and weighs more than 13 pounds, you're virtually assured of it.

Concerned that your baby will begin to suffer nutritionally, especially if she has been consuming a significant amount of milk at night? Not to worry. Studies show that there is no decrease in total milk intake over a 24-hour period after nighttime feedings are eliminated. The baby simply makes up for the missing midnight snack by eating more during the day.

If you're lucky, nature may solve the problem for you, as the laws of evolution determine that the mother's need for sleep has become more critical than the child's need for around-the-clock sustenance. My own mother, Jean Nicholls, claims that this is the process through which all seven of her children began to sleep through the night. "With each baby, there came a time, usually around age 3 or 4 months, when I was simply so exhausted that I wouldn't hear the baby cry in the middle of the night. Actually, I probably heard him on a subconscious level, because I'd always have some perfectly logical dream about why it was okay for that baby to be fussing—and so I'd go right on sleeping," she explains. "I'd awaken at dawn and realize with horror that I'd never gotten up to give the baby a bottle. So I'd run to the nursery, afraid the poor little thing would be on the verge of starvation, and find him or her asleep in the crib in perfect contentment. At that point, I figured the baby didn't really need to eat at night anymore."

When Mother Nature doesn't step in to save the day, however, you'll need to take matters into your own hands. There are several methods for doing that. Choose the one that's best suited to your own personal parenting style.

THE COLD-TURKEY APPROACH

Some parents feel comfortable with this method once they recognize that there is no longer any physiological need for their baby to be fed at night. Simply put, you just say no to any and all future demands for nighttime feeding. You may do this by staying out of the nursery altogether, or by checking on the baby periodically to reassure her of your presence but not to offer a breast or bottle.

"When Leah was 7 months old, it occurred to me that the only reason she was still waking up twice a night to nurse was because I was making myself available to her. She weighed close to 20 pounds and was as tubby as the Michelin Man, so she certainly didn't need those extra feedings," explains Amy Marz, mother of two girls. "I decided to go cold turkey. The first and second nights, Leah screamed for almost 2 hours. The third and fourth nights, the wailing went on for perhaps half an hour. And that was it. By the fifth night, Leah was sleeping through without the slightest bit of fussing."

Wasn't it hard to listen to all that howling? "Sure it was," Amy admits. "But my philosophy is, as long as my parental expectations are reasonable, I don't need to feel guilty about enforcing the rules. And I think it's reasonable to expect a 7-month-old to sleep through the night."

The cold-turkey approach can also be quick and effective for a baby who wakes and cries for the breast or bottle but who actually consumes only a small amount of milk. Marey Oakes's daughter Grace habitually did just that. "Grace would nurse for just a few minutes before falling back to sleep—not long enough to get more than an ounce or two of milk. I knew she was using me as a pacifier more than as a provider of nourishment," says Marey. Grace was 11 months old by this time, and was virtually weaned except for this nighttime snacking. "The way the situation finally got resolved was that I went away for a long weekend, leaving the kids home with my husband. And by the time I got back, Grace's nighttime nursing habit was history."

THE GRADUAL WEANING APPROACH

Many parents, and many experts, too, are ill at ease with the cold-turkey approach, preferring a more gradual method for eliminating nighttime feedings. "Even if a baby is eating out of habit rather than nutritional need, it would be cruel to suddenly withhold all food at night," says Dr. Ferber. You know the baby no longer requires those calories, but he doesn't know it—and while he's certainly not starving, he really does feel hungry. So since you were partly responsible for his developing the midnight snacking habit, he'll appreciate your help in breaking it.

Step 1. Space out daytime feedings more. You may reason that by feeding your baby more often during the day, you can fill her up enough so that she won't be hungry at night. But in fact, the opposite is true. A baby who gets used to eating frequently during the day consumes only a small amount at any given time. She becomes a snacker, and she wants those snacks to be constantly available no matter what the hour.

Instead, you should stretch out the intervals between daytime feedings, so your baby gets used to taking in more milk at one time. This way, she'll learn to be satisfied with fewer but larger feedings. What's a reasonable goal? "By age 4 months, you can aim for four meals each day for a formula-fed baby, or five meals a day if you're breast-feeding," suggests Dr. Barton D. Schmitt.

Of course, if you currently feed your baby every hour, you can't expect to jump instantly into a 4-hour feeding schedule. But you can increase the waiting intervals gradually, 30 minutes at a time. Once your baby accepts being fed every 1½ hours, stretch the wait to 2 hours. Work your way up until your baby's accustomed to waiting 3 to 4 hours between meals.

It's not easy to delay a feeding when you've got a hungry baby on your hands, but it can be done. When the baby awakens from his nap, change his diaper slowly. Then take him for a walk or play with him; if he's well entertained, he may forget about food for a while. If he seems to have a strong need to suck, you might offer him a pacifier or help him find his thumb. Avoid holding him in the feeding position during the 30-minute wait, or he's likely to feel extremely frustrated when he finds no food is forthcoming.

Remember, too, that a baby's cry is not always a signal of hunger. He may be bored, lonely, gassy, overheated, overstimulated, or overtired. He doesn't need food; he needs you to figure out why he's unhappy, and fix it. "Don't let feeding become a pacifier," urges Dr. Schmitt. "For every time you nurse your baby, there should be four or five times that you snuggle him without nursing."

Step 2. Space out nighttime feedings more. Once the daytime feedings are on a more acceptable schedule, you can gradually start to reduce the number of times you feed the baby at night. To do this, increase the waiting interval between nighttime feedings by 30 minutes at a time.

When your baby wakes up too soon for a feeding, try getting her back to sleep with soft, soothing murmurs and some pats on the back. If whimpering turns to wailing, comfort her without picking her up for as long as possible. Once you feel you must pick her up, avoid holding her in the customary feeding position. A breast-fed baby may find this wait less irksome if Dad handles the 30-minute stalling routine. Otherwise, it's extremely aggravating to the baby to know that Mommy's breast is right there next to her, yet she's inexplicably being denied access.

Another option is to reduce the amount of milk

given during each nighttime feeding. This can be done instead of, or in addition to, the stretching procedure described above. "To begin, cut back by an ounce or two on the amount of milk in the bottle. If you're nursing, reduce the time the baby is at each breast, or offer only one breast per feeding," suggests Dr. Jodi Mindell.

What to do once only a minimal amount of milk is being consumed during a nighttime feeding? Some experts recommend eliminating that feeding altogether, either by letting the baby fuss until she falls back to sleep, or by visiting her periodically to reassure her of your presence, but without picking her up. Other experts suggest offering the baby a bit of water instead, on the theory that she'll soon decide it's not worth waking up for water, and will simply start to sleep through with no further complaining. If you're a nursing mother, you might prefer to have your partner offer the water bottle. Otherwise, it can be painful for you to hold the crying baby without nursing her, since your breasts may be uncomfortably full.

There is one situation in which the gradual weaning approach will not work—with a baby who habitually wakes and cries to be fed, but then drinks only an ounce from her bottle or nurses only briefly before dropping off again. The reason it won't work is that this baby is not a true trained night feeder, since she's obviously not really hungry. Instead, she's what's called a trained night crier. Solutions to this problem are offered later in this chapter, in the section called Quieting the "Trained Night Crier" (see page 91).

Should you let your baby feed herself a bottle? To many parents, this seems like a reasonable solution.

By the time a baby is 6 to 8 months old, he may be able to hold his own bottle—so why not simply prepare one in advance, place it in his eager hands when he cries at 2 A.M., and head straight back to bed yourself?

Though this sounds like an easy way around the problem, it's in fact potentially quite harmful. For one thing, it can do severe damage to a baby's developing teeth even before they erupt. Milk that pools around the gums and lingers there for much of the night can cause a form of tooth decay known as baby-bottle caries. Fluid in the mouth can also find its way up into the nose and ears, increasing the risk of ear infections. Worst of all, there's a very real danger that the baby could choke to death if part of the nipple breaks off and lodges in his throat.

If your baby is already a nighttime self-feeder, you need to put a stop to this. You can try the cold-turkey method outlined on pages 83–84, perhaps substituting a pacifier for the bottle. Or you can start again to hold the baby for his nighttime feedings, then implement the gradual weaning approach.

―――――――――――――――― ✳ ――――――――――――――――

The Great Debate About Solid Foods

Grandma may tell you your 3-month-old (or even your 3-week-old) would sleep through the night if only you'd give her some solid food. She'll swear it worked for her.

But before you mix that formula with barley flakes, consider this: there is no evidence that feeding an infant solid food at bedtime postpones nighttime hunger or prolongs sleep. Dr. Wolfson explains, "Scientific studies have found no correlation between the age at which babies are fed solid foods and the age at which they sleep through night." Some experts find that the more likely correlation seems to be with weight. Once a baby reaches about 12 pounds, he's more apt to sleep through the night no matter what his diet.

An infant under the age of 4 months does not benefit from being fed cereal, fruit, or other solids, because breastmilk or an iron-fortified formula meets all her nutritional needs. On the contrary, premature introduction of solid foods can trigger food intolerances and allergies. The resulting discomfort is hardly the thing to promote a good night's sleep.

Still think you'd like to try solids? Then get your pediatrician's okay first, start slow, and back off immediately if your baby shows any signs of intolerance.

AGE FLAG: 1 TO 3 YEARS

With an older child who drinks well from a cup during the day yet still insists on having a bottle in her crib at night, your best bet is to persuade her to give up bottles altogether. "Help your child make the emotional break from her bottle," suggests Dr. Mindell. "Tell her that if she leaves the bottles out for the Bottle Fairy to take away, the fairy will leave a gift for her in return. Or you can help her pack the bottles up in a box and pretend to mail them to the hungry babies in a poorer country."

Or you can be on the lookout for opportune moments to implement a new no-more-bottles policy. "I'd been trying for months to break Chip of his nighttime bottle habit. He was almost 2 years old, and I figured enough was enough already. But no success," says Judy Dooley, a mother of four. "Then one evening, the funniest thing happened. We were going to my brother's house, and I thought I'd better bring along a bottle in case the party went late and I wanted to put Chip to bed over there. But as we were driving along the highway on our way to the party, Chip—who was playing with the empty bottle—accidentally dropped the bottle out the car window. That night when he asked for his bottle, I reminded him that it was gone. To my relief, he accepted this and settled back down pretty easily. Of course after that, I pretended the lost bottle had been our only bottle. I secretly got rid of Chip's other bottles, and after a night or two of just a little fussing, Chip forgot all about them."

How to Handle Your Toddler's Nighttime Hunger

AGE FLAG: 1 YEAR AND UP

Suppose your youngster has been sleeping through the night for months or even years, yet suddenly he's waking up each night and begging for a midnight snack. This is not a good pattern to get into. "If he gets proper nutrition during the day, and your pediatrician verifies that his growth is normal, there's no reason why your toddler should need to eat at night," says Dr. Mindell. To put a halt to the habit, first try to figure out what's triggering it.

• Perhaps he eats dinner too early, so that by bedtime his tummy is empty. After a cycle of sleep or two, he wakes up, feels his stomach rumbling, and wants a bite to eat. The fix: schedule dinner for a later time or offer him a snack before bed.

- Some youngsters are so tired by evening that they eat very little supper, then wake up hungry in the middle of the night. Try giving him an earlier dinner so he's alert enough to eat a full meal. Also, offer him a glass of milk at bedtime.

- What if hunger wakes him at 4 A.M. rather than midnight? It may be that he's accustomed to eating first thing in the morning, but now instead of waiting till 6 A.M. for that cereal, his tummy's demanding breakfast 1 or 2 hours earlier. Take a two-pronged approach. First, give him a snack at bedtime so he doesn't wake up ravenous. Second, start delaying his breakfast for an hour after he wakes up, to help break the association between rising and immediately eating.

If none of these tactics solve the problem, Dr. Mindell suggests taking a cold-turkey approach. "Simply tell the child, 'No more food during the night.' He'll quickly learn to make up for those lost calories by eating more during the day."

QUIETING THE "TRAINED NIGHT CRIER"

AGE FLAG: 6 MONTHS AND UP

"My little boy, James, is almost a year old and still he doesn't sleep through the night," I griped to a woman I happened to meet at a party. "He wakes up every night around 3 A.M., and I have to rock him and nurse him until he falls back to sleep."

"Does he nurse for a long time at night?" she asked.

"No, just for a couple minutes. That's what makes it so maddening, because it's obvious he's not really hungry."

"Do you rock him and nurse him to sleep at bedtime, too? And before his naps during the day?" she inquired.

"Sure. It's the easiest way to settle him down. Works every time," I answered.

"Well then, that's your problem. He thinks the only way to fall asleep is to have his mommy's arms around him and her breast in his mouth. So when he wakes up at night and doesn't have those things, he cries until you give them back to him."

To me, this was a major revelation. I'd never before heard about sleep associations—the conditions under which a person is accustomed to fall asleep, and without which it becomes difficult to drop off—yet the concept seemed inarguably logical. Within a week, I'd found a way to free my son and myself from his overly dependent sleep associations, and we both started sleeping a lot better. (How'd I do it? That method, and many others, are described later in this chapter.)

A trained night crier is a child over the age of 6 months who wakes up in the middle of the night and cannot go back to sleep without some sort of help from you. That help can take a variety of forms. Does your child demand that you rock him, stroke him, sing to him? Does he want you to pace the floor with him in your arms, or put him in the car and drive around town? Does he insist on sucking a breast or bottle, yet actually consumes almost nothing? If you've answered yes to any of these questions, you've got a trained night crier in your family.

The Problem with Parent-Dependent
Sleep Associations

Chapter Two explained in detail the concept of sleep associations—that a person grows used to having specific conditions met when falling asleep, and when those conditions are not met, it can be extremely difficult to get to sleep.

Sleep associations come into play not just at bedtime, but also any time a person wakes up in the middle of the night. Remember, as we discussed in Chapter One, everyone does wake up momentarily several times each night. We may look around a bit, assure ourselves that all is well, then roll over and go right back to sleep without leaving in our memory any lasting imprint of that brief awakening.

But if when we awaken we find that all is not as we expected it to be—why is that hall light on? why is my pillow on the floor? why is that faucet dripping?—we probably feel compelled to correct the situation. Turn off that light, pick up that pillow, give that leaky faucet another turn. That done, we can finally go back to sleep.

For a baby, the same thing occurs. Suppose that every night at 8 P.M. you rock your baby and she falls easily into peaceful slumber. You lay her in her crib, go about the evening's business, and then go to bed yourself. But after completing a few cycles of sleep, the baby wakes up, a perfectly normal thing to do. She looks around a bit to assure herself that all is well. And what does she find? That all is most decidedly not well. Where are the arms that are supposed to be enfolding her? Where is that rocking sensation that's supposed to soothe her tiny nerves? Where is that comforting scent, the one that means Mommy is near? No wonder she can't go back to sleep. Her whole universe has been altered. All that is cozy and familiar is gone, and in its place there is only a strange, still solitude. It doesn't matter to her that it's midnight or 3 A.M. She is going to express her dismay in the only way she knows how—with angry screams or piteous cries—until you come and make the world right again.

There is one type of trained night crier who follows a slightly different pattern. He goes to sleep easily and independently at bedtime, without requiring any active participation from you. But when he awakens at 2 A.M., he wants company. He calls out for you, and you come; he reaches up for you, and you pick him up; he bestows his most beguiling "play with me now" smile, and you play with him. Perhaps it begins by accident one night when he really isn't very tired. Then the next night when he awakens, he remembers how much fun he had with Mommy or Daddy the night before, so he cries out for you again, and again you respond. And then he, little party animal, is hooked on the nighttime-is-funtime habit—and so are you.

Can you simply bide your time and hope your baby outgrows her trained night crying? You can, but you'll probably be disappointed. Studies show that nighttime wakings continue to be a problem with up to 25 percent of toddlers and 15 percent of preschoolers. The particulars will change, of course. She'll no longer cry helplessly in her crib; she'll pop right out of bed and walk out of her room. She won't demand a bottle; she'll ask for a glass of water or a grilled cheese sandwich. She won't need to be rocked in her rocking chair; she'll just climb into your bed for a snuggle. She won't be content with a quick run-through of "This Little Piggy"; she'll want you to break out the storybooks or the Candyland gameboard. She'll have graduated from the ranks of the trained night criers, and entered into the big-kid corps called trained night wakers.

So instead of adopting a laissez-faire attitude, you're better off nipping the problem in the bud right now. Fortunately, there are a variety of approaches you can take. Choose the one that seems best suited to your particular situation, your child's temperament, and your own parenting philosophy. Or combine two or more of the methods to create your own custom-designed solution.

THE ROOT-OF-THE-PROBLEM APPROACH: GO BACK AND FIX THE BEDTIME PROBLEM FIRST

Maybe you don't think you have a bedtime problem. You're content to spend the time it takes each evening at 8 P.M. to nurse your baby to sleep, to sing her songs until slumber comes, to scratch her back until she dozes off. But ask yourself: are you equally content to nurse, sing, and scratch all over again at midnight and at 2 A.M. and at 4 A.M.? If not, you probably ought to re-evaluate the bedtime routine. Dr. Mindell reports, "Studies show that children whose parents are routinely present when they fall asleep at bedtime have far more frequent disruptive night wakings."

Turn back to Chapter Two. Review the section on Sleep Associations: How They Affect a Child's Ability to Fall Asleep, and implement the bedtime policies outlined there. There are several compelling reasons to do this. "For one thing, you'll find it less stressful to initiate a new routine at the child's bedtime, when you are still wide awake. You'll have more energy for sticking with the method until it works. But if you skip the bedtime step and just tackle the nighttime problem, you'll be so exhausted and desperate for sleep yourself that you may give in to whatever the child wants, just so he'll quiet down and let you go back to bed," warns Dr. Mindell.

Important reason number two is that once the overly dependent sleep associations that surround bedtime are broken, the disruptive nighttime awakenings may simply disappear. "In 80 percent of cases, letting the child learn how to fall asleep on her own at bedtime spontaneously resolves the nighttime problem as well," Dr. Mindell points out. In other words, you may never have to address the 2 A.M. situation directly, because there's a very good chance the problem will simply evaporate.

In establishing a new bedtime routine for your child, your primary aim is to extricate yourself from her going-to-sleep process. That means you'll no longer allow her to fall asleep at your breast or over a bottle, in your arms or with your hand on her back, to the sound of your voice or to the motion of your body as you walk her around and around the room. A variety of means for achieving this are described in detail in Chapter Two.

But simply removing yourself from the final bedtime scene is not enough. You must also consider all the other elements that may currently contribute to her sleep-association problem. Your goal is for her new bedtime environment to duplicate exactly the environment in which she will find herself when she awakens spontaneously during the night. Will your baby be spending the entire night in her bouncer, playpen, or swing? Certainly not, so don't let her fall asleep there after dinner, thinking you can transfer her into the crib later on. Will the hall light be off at midnight? Then don't leave it on when you put the baby to bed at 8 P.M. Will the nursery door be open at 2 o'clock in the morning? If so, don't shut it behind you after you bestow that final bedtime kiss. Will the sound of the television waft from the family room to the baby's bedroom at 4 A.M.? Highly unlikely—so don't let it filter in while your baby's falling asleep in the evening.

If you're one of the unlucky ones for whom a correction in the bedtime routine does not automatically eliminate the disruptive nighttime wakings, take heart. You still have many options left.

THE WAIT-AND-SEE APPROACH

In describing the wait-and-see approach, I don't mean to wait for weeks or months or years while praying the problem goes away on its own. I mean that rather than rush to the child's side at the first whimper, you can wait a moment or two to see if he settles down on his own.

Remember, as discussed in Chapter One, a child has more REM sleep than an adult does, so he's bound to move around and make more noise in his sleep. Nonetheless, he is asleep—and he's more likely to stay asleep if his parents refrain from dashing into his room to check on him every half-hour. On the other hand, when each semialert period is reinforced with a feeding, a lullaby, or a lot of hugs, the baby gets the message that waking fully is a good thing, because it results in a reward. His natural sleep rhythms are disturbed, and he loses the ability to soothe himself back to sleep.

Not sure how long to wait before checking up on a whimpering babe? Try counting to 100 slowly to give those squawks a chance to subside. Or put your sleep diary to double use now: to record your youngster's sleep/wake patterns, and as a stalling tactic to force yourself to stay put for a few minutes. Dr. Madansky shares this story: "One mother reported to me that her baby awoke 14 times each night. I suspected that, in truth, the well-meaning mom was rushing in every time the child made the slightest twitch or grunt, even though such sounds and movements are characteristic of normal REM sleep. I suggested that she keep a sleep log. The result: by the time she had turned on her light and entered the date and time of the supposed 'awakening' in the log, the baby usually would have settled back to sleep already."

This method is so simple and effort-free that it should probably be used each time your child awakens, no matter what other techniques you may decide to try.

THE IGNORE-IT METHOD

AGE FLAG: 6 MONTHS TO 2½ YEARS

The ignore-it method is essentially the same as the cry-it-out method described in Chapter Two as an option for handling bedtime protests, and is most effective with a child who cannot yet climb out of her crib. In brief, when the child wakes up in the middle of the night and cries or calls out for you, go to her room to make sure that nothing is really wrong. Quickly verify that the child is neither sick nor in pain nor particularly afraid, then leave. Offer no kisses, no stories, no soothing—nothing that would represent a reward for the child's awakening. And then proceed to ignore the child, no matter how long or how loudly she cries. Does it really work? Yes, and usually quite quickly.

"My twins had been sleeping through the night for many months. Then one night, when they were 9 months old, they woke up at 3 A.M. and started to scream and carry on. Since they'd never acted like that before, I was worried that something was terribly wrong. I ran to them, soothed them, rocked them till my arms were sore, and finally they settled down. Then the same thing happened again the next night. And the next, and the next, and the next," says Lisa Cool, mother of three girls. "After a month of this, I'd had enough. My husband and I didn't like the term *crying it out,* so we coined our own phrase: *howl therapy.* We decided that when the twins started to cry, we would check on them once to make sure they were okay, and then we would just ignore them. The first night they cried for over an hour, the second night for half an hour, the third night for 10 minutes. And after that, they never bothered to cry at night again. I admit it was pretty grim that first night, but, boy, was it worth it!"

Implement your own version of howl therapy at a

time when your child is feeling well and no other major changes are taking place in his life.

AGE FLAG: 1 TO 2½ YEARS

If your crib-bound child is old enough to talk, your task may be a bit harder. "The ignoring technique can shake the resolve of even the most determined parent," admits Dr. Schaefer. "To bolster your chances of success, before you use this tactic, plan how you'll handle the stress of hearing your child cry out, 'Mommy, I need you. Daddy, help me.'"

AGE FLAG: 2 YEARS AND UP

The ignore-it approach is trickier, too, when used with a child who can climb out of her crib or who already sleeps in a regular bed, because there are no physical restraints to keep her in her room. Details on how to handle such a situation are discussed in Chapter Five.

If you cannot resist responding to your child's cries or heartrending appeals, or if you feel it would be wrong to do so, the ignore-it method is not for you. Instead, move on to one of the approaches outlined below.

THE REASSURING APPROACH

AGE FLAG: 6 MONTHS TO 2½ YEARS

The nighttime version of the reassuring approach is virtually identical to the bedtime version detailed in Chapter Two. It's appropriate for children over the age of 6 months who still sleep in a crib. Following is a short review. When your child wakes up and cries in the middle of the night, wait 5 minutes before responding. Then go to her room and, without picking her up or turning on the light, verbally reassure her that all is well. Linger no more than 1 minute, then leave the room. If the child keeps on crying, wait 10 minutes, return to her room and briefly reassure her again, then leave. If the crying still continues, wait 15 minutes before returning to her. Repeat this waiting/reassuring cycle every 15 minutes until the child falls back to sleep during one of the intervals in which you are not in her room. The second night, wait 10 minutes before responding for the first time, and stretch each waiting interval for an additional 5 minutes.

If you're uncomfortable with the suggested length of the intervals, start with shorter waiting periods—perhaps 1 minute, then 2, then 3—and gradually work your way up. Whatever length waiting interval you select, keep the reassurance portion of the method short. Maintain a calm but businesslike demeanor. Don't reprimand the child for disturbing you, but don't offer any positive reinforcement, either—no hugs, no games, no stories. Your intention is to show the child that you are there so he feels safe, but not to give in to his demands for attention. This is the method I used with my son, James, who at 11 months was still waking me at 3 A.M. every night. The first night was pretty horrible—but by the fourth night, peace reigned.

Some children protest sleep training by using weapons that are hard for parents to fight. "My wife and I had agreed to try this method of periodically visiting our son's room, but otherwise to let him cry. The sound of his screaming set our nerves so on edge that we couldn't even think of climbing back into bed ourselves. So we stood outside his closed door, anxiously counting down the seconds until we could go in to him again," recalls Abe Carlton (not his real name). "Finally, it was time. We threw open the door, dashed in, and found our baby boy covered with vomit. We felt horribly guilty, of course, so we cleaned him up and brought him into bed with us." The next night, Abe and his wife decided to give it another shot. "Again, we were standing outside his door waiting for it to be time to go in. Suddenly, we heard this unmistakable sound. We ran in, and sure enough, he'd thrown up again, so we threw in the towel. We felt there was no way we could win that battle, not against a kid who fights that dirty."

Abe needn't have surrendered altogether, however. Dr. Mindell explains, "Don't be too alarmed if your child vomits from crying hard. It's actually a fairly common occurrence. As long as she shows no other signs of illness, it doesn't mean the child is sick. It just means she has figured out that throwing up is the most effective way to get Mom and Dad to rush in and pick her up, make a big fuss over her, and give her whatever she wants."

So what's a parent to do? Dr. Mindell answers, "Before bedtime, lay out an extra pair of clean pajamas and cover the mattress with two sheets, one on top of the other. If the child vomits during the night, matter-of-factly change her pajamas and strip off the dirty sheet on top to expose the clean one underneath. Put the child straight to bed, say good night, leave the room, and get right back into the sleep-training routine." Once you succeed in eliminating your child's disruptive awakenings, those few extra loads of laundry will seem a small price to have paid for the undisturbed slumber that will be yours.

THE LAY-DOWN-THE-LAW (NICELY) TECHNIQUE

AGE FLAG: 2 YEARS AND UP

Once a kid is old enough to climb out of his crib or sleep in a regular bed, it becomes logistically difficult to enforce the reassuring approach. At this point, you'll do better to lay down the law, gently but firmly. Here's a sample script:

PARENT: Timmy, we need to make a new rule. I need for you to stay quietly in your bed at night, instead of calling out for me or coming into my room.

CHILD: I can't help it. Sometimes I just wake up and I can't get back to sleep.

PARENT: I'm not saying you're not allowed to wake up— everybody wakes up at night sometimes—but I am saying you may not disturb me. Nighttime is for sleeping. You need your rest, and I need mine. When you wake me up at night, I feel tired and grumpy the next day. I'll tell you what. We'll make a star chart. For each night you stay quietly in your own bed, you'll earn a star. When you've earned five stars, I'll buy you a new video.

(Later that night, after the child has awakened and called out for his father:)

CHILD: Dad, I just can't fall back to sleep. Won't you stay here and talk to me awhile?

PARENT: No. This is not the time to talk or play. Go back to sleep. I know you can do it. (Leaves room.)

(In the morning, a few days later:)

PARENT: Tim, I'm really proud of you for not waking me up last night. Let's paste a star on your chart now. It won't be long before you earn that new video.

This kind of conversation aims to accomplish several things. It clearly explains the new rules: no crying, no calling out, no coming into the parent's room. It offers the child a simple explanation for the new policy—that nighttime is for sleeping and everyone needs his or her rest. When the youngster fails to comply, his father reminds him of the rule, without harsh reprimands but also without any signs of warmth or affection that could reinforce the night wakings. The father expresses confidence in his son's ability to exercise self-control. The star chart and verbal praise provide positive reinforcement as the boy makes progress, and the promise of a small prize further motivates the child to cooperate.

Strategies for Parents Who Can't Bear to Hear a Baby Cry

There are those parents who find almost any crying intolerable. Perhaps they live in an apartment or condominium, and the child's howls bother the other tenants. Perhaps one spouse insists that his sleep not be disturbed, or suffers greatly when it is. Perhaps the parents are just too tenderhearted to listen to their child scream, even if they know it will probably end after a few nights.

"I'm so tired of getting out of bed at 2 A.M. when my baby boy cries. At 7 months, he's certainly old enough to sleep through the night, and I'd be willing to ignore his cries until he learned to do so," says Marey Oakes. "In fact, I usually don't even wake up when the baby cries in the middle of the night. The problem is, my husband Michael wakes up at the first peep, and he can't go back to sleep until the baby's quiet again. And when Michael doesn't get enough rest, he gets a bad migraine. He never insists that I get up to comfort the baby, of course—he's too considerate to do that—but I know how much he'll suffer if I don't."

If you're in a similar situation, the sleep-training methods described in this section may help. But be forewarned: these methods require a lot more participation on your part, and may take much longer to succeed than the approaches outlined previously.

THE BEDSIDE-REASSURANCE TECHNIQUE

The bedside-reassurance approach is worth a try if your youngster typically wakes up three or more times during the night. It's easier to implement with a tot who sleeps in a crib, but may also be successful with an older child who sleeps in a bed.

To prepare, place a cot in the child's room. During the night, when the child wakes up and cries for the first time, go into her room and reassure the child that all is well, but do not take her out of her bed. Then lie down on the cot and sleep there for the rest of the night. Each time your child awakens, speak to her from your cot and quietly reassure her: "Mommy's here; everything's fine. Go back to sleep now."

There's a threefold purpose to this. "The parent is reassured that the child is fine; the child is reassured by the parent's presence; and the parent models good sleep behavior for the child," explains Dr. Madansky. "The theory is that, within two or three nights, the child will be feeling comfortable and secure enough at night that her pattern of constant awakenings will start to give way to better sleep habits."

Here's the caveat: after three nights on the cot, the parent must move out of the child's room. At that point, if the child awakens and cries at night, you simply go to her doorway and reassure her verbally—and hope that by now she's better able to soothe herself back to sleep.

Does it really work? Sometimes. "Most kids do show measurable improvement after the three nights, and some are able to sleep through," says Dr. Madansky.

There's one type of child with whom this method will not work: the kid who becomes enraged when his mother or father refuses to take him out of the crib, even though that parent is clearly visible on the cot. When the parent's presence causes the child to scream in frustration rather than to feel reassured enough to settle down, a different method must be tried.

STEP-BY-STEP BEHAVIOR MODIFICATION

AGE FLAG: 6 MONTHS AND UP

Try the step-by-step approach with a trained night crier who's accustomed to having a parent provide several different forms of soothing, either simultaneously or sequentially. The technique can be used whether the child sleeps in a crib or bed. Start with your sleep log. Record the time the child goes to bed, the time at which she wakes during the night, and every single step you take to get her back to sleep. Now look closely at your role. How many different soothing tactics do you use? How can you gradually involve yourself less?

Suppose each time your child wakes, you pick her up, rock her in a chair, offer her some milk, play a quick game of Pop Goes the Weasel, and then sing to her until she sleeps once more. For her, what fun! No wonder she likes to wake you up at night—but that's not much fun for you. "Your goal is to reduce the fun factor gradually enough that you don't elicit any loud complaints from the child, but quickly enough that you do not become discouraged by slow progress," Dr. Madansky says.

Start by eliminating one or two of your customary soothing strategies. Can you skip the game of Pop Goes the Weasel without your child taking much notice? Then do so. Now tone down the rest of the routine. Substitute water for the milk, then cut out the drink altogether. Change your songs to a soft murmur, then to no sound at all. Hold her in your lap without rocking for a few nights, then just hold her hand while she stays in bed.

Once the child has accepted these changes, slowly remove yourself from the scene. Instead of sitting on her bed, sit in a chair next to the bed. Each night move the chair closer to the door. Then try simply standing in the doorway to offer a brief word of comfort. Eventually, your child will decide that this small reward is not worth the effort of waking up fully, and she'll simply go back to sleep.

THE BEAT-HIM-TO-THE-PUNCH APPROACH

AGE FLAG: 2 YEARS AND UP

More formally known as scheduled awakenings, the beat-him-to-the-punch technique involves waking the child yourself before he has a chance to wake you. It works best with children who already sleep in a regular bed and so cannot be forced to stay in their crib. In preparation, keep a sleep diary for 7 days, noting when your child goes to sleep and when he awakens. "You'll probably find a pattern, not necessarily based on the clock, but rather on the length of the period that elapses between the time the child falls asleep and the time he awakens," says Vaughn I. Rickert, Psy.D., associate professor of pediatrics at the University of Arkansas for Medical Sciences in Little Rock. For instance, suppose the child typically awakens 2½ hours after falling asleep. If he goes to bed at 8:30 on any given night, you can expect to hear from him around 11:00; when his bedtime is delayed until 9:30, you can anticipate an awakening at midnight.

Assume, for simplicity's sake, that your child usually goes to sleep at 8:30 and wakes at 11:00. Your job, for the next three nights, is to wake him up 30 minutes before you expect him to awaken on his own—in this case, around 10:30 P.M. Dr. Rickert explains, "After you rouse the child, do whatever you would normally do when his waking is spontaneous, but do it a little less. Instead of picking him up out of bed, just rub his back; instead of telling him a story, just murmur softly. The idea is to get him somewhat alert, but not wide awake. Then let the child go back to sleep. Most likely, he will sleep straight through his customary awakening time."

On the fourth night, delay the scheduled awakening for half an hour; instead of rousing the child at 10:30, wake him at 11:00. Do this for three consecutive nights. Then postpone the scheduled awakening for another 30 minutes, so you're rousing the child at 11:30. Follow this pattern—rousing him at the same time for three nights, then delaying for another half-hour—until the scheduled awakening is occurring at 4 o'clock in the morning. After three nights of waking the child at 4 A.M., stop waking him altogether. If the method has succeeded, he'll simply sleep through till morning.

What if your child typically wakes more than once during the night? You must schedule an awakening 30 minutes prior to each anticipated spontaneous awakening, then gradually delay so that each awakening occurs later and later at night. Eventually, all awakenings will be eliminated. This makes the process more complicated, of course, but does not necessarily render it ineffective.

The hardest part about using this method is getting out of bed yourself for those scheduled awakenings that are to occur at 2 or 3 A.M. But, Dr. Rickert assures, if you force yourself to stick with it, the method most likely will succeed. Why it succeeds is a bit of a mystery, however. "It could be that by rousing the child from a deeper stage of sleep, you give him practice in falling back to sleep when he has a strong physiological inclination to do so," Dr. Rickert suggests.

Compared to other sleep-training methods that target the night crier, this one admittedly takes the longest—usually about a month—and requires a lot more effort on the part of the parent. But it involves virtually no crying. If that's your number-one priority, the beat-him-to-the-punch approach could be a perfect solution for you.

Still feeling conflicted about using sleep-training methods to deal with disruptive nighttime wakings? Don't let unwarranted feelings of guilt get in the way. Sure, you'll be happier once you're no longer forced out of bed in the middle of the night—but your child will benefit immensely, too. As long as you're acting out of love, you won't go wrong no matter which approach you use.

✳ FOUR

*Night Frights: What to Do
When Kids Get Scared*

Clare Gunther tossed beneath the blankets. She needed to get some rest, but sleep was slow to come. She thought of the work deadlines approaching too fast, of the argument she'd had with her second-grade son at dinner, of how her husband's business trips seemed to take him farther and farther from home. Finally, fitfully, she dozed off.

She awoke to the sound of a terrified scream. Annie! Clare dashed into her daughter's room. Eyes open wide and sobbing with fright, 3-year-old Anne could scarcely choke out the words. "He tried to take me away with him. He came through my window and grabbed me and said I'd never see my mommy again!"

"Who did?" asked Clare, holding the child tightly against her chest.

"Peter Pan," Anne wailed. "He wanted to take me to Never Land."

If you haven't yet been confronted by your child's nighttime fears, chances are that you will be someday soon. Virtually all children experience some type of night fright, whether it's triggered by separation anxiety, childhood phobias, nightmares, or a phenomenon known as night terrors. Fortunately, there's much you can do to help your child feel safer and less afraid as she faces her nighttime fears—so you'll both sleep better.

How Separation Anxiety Can Affect Sleep

AGE FLAG: 6 MONTHS TO 2 YEARS

Many people think of separation anxiety as a daytime problem. It's what makes a 10-month-old crawl over and clutch your ankle when you try to walk from the playroom to the kitchen. It's what makes a 16-month-old insist on sitting in your lap while you use the toilet, instead of allowing you a few private moments behind a closed door. It's what makes a 2-year-old sob or scream when you drop him off at nursery school.

But in fact, what separation anxiety affects most is a child's sleep. "A child with separation anxiety typically learns to cope with her daily activities—to play, chatter, eat well—even when Mom's not around. But long after she's adjusted to daytime separations, she may still have trouble at night," explains Tiffany Field, Ph.D., professor of psychology, pediatrics, and psychiatry at the University of Miami School of Medicine. She clings to you when you try to lay her in her crib, shrieks as you leave the nursery. Slumber, when it comes, is lighter and more restless. And even if she had been sleeping through the night for months, she now wakes in the wee hours and cries out for you to come to her.

Think such behavior portends a life of obsessive dependence? Not so. Separation anxiety is a normal developmental phase during which a child fears being apart from his primary caregiver. Typically, it first appears between 6 and 12 months of age, and peaks within a few months after the first birthday. "It begins when a baby becomes aware of his parents as individuals separate from himself, and realizes that being separate involves some danger," says Dr. Charles E. Schaefer. "What's more, he cannot yet imagine where you are if you're not in sight. When you leave, it appears that you've gone forever." Bedtime brings all of your baby's anxieties to the fore because going to sleep means letting go of you and trusting that you'll still be there in the morning.

AGE FLAG: 2 TO 3 YEARS

Some babies quickly outgrow their separation fears; for others, the anxiety persists for several years. It's not uncommon for a 2- or 3-year-old, panicked at the thought of being apart from her parents all night, to plead, "Sleep with me, Mommy," or "Let me stay in the living room with you."

Of course, there are many other reasons why a baby or toddler might resist going to bed or cry in the middle of the night. How can you be sure you're dealing with separation anxiety and not some other sleep problem? "If she always quiets down the moment you take one step inside her room, that's a strong indication of anxiety," notes Dr. Richard Ferber. She'll also cry whenever you leave her during the day, not only at bedtime. Another clue: her clinging worsens following an upsetting event such as getting lost momentarily in a store or park, changing caregivers, the birth of a new sibling, or a mother's return to work. For example, my son James's separation anxiety surfaced right after I doubled the number of hours I devoted each week to my part-time work. And of course, a major trauma such as an illness or death in the family, or her parents' divorce, will almost certainly increase the anxiety a child feels when apart from her parents.

Easing Separation Anxiety–Related Sleep Problems

AGE FLAG: 6 MONTHS TO 3 YEARS

You may find that bedtime separations go more smoothly when your youngster receives plenty of loving physical contact during his waking hours. If your baby is still small enough, try carrying her around the house in a Snugli, sling, or backpack. Playing peek-a-boo gives baby a chance to practice separating from you momentarily by covering his eyes. Older children accomplish the same end with games of hide-and-seek, and by being sent into another room to fetch a toy or article of clothing. Toddlers and preschoolers also benefit from talking about their worries, though it's best to restrict such discussions to the daytime so that bedtime worrying won't become a habit.

No matter what your child's age, it's also important that *you* not appear overly anxious about separations,

Dr. Field cautions. "Whenever you take leave of your child, do it calmly. Don't act worried or sad, and don't drag out your goodbyes. When you return, do so not with desperate hugs and kisses, but with a smile."

As for what you can do at night to help a child through this anxious phase, expert opinion varies. Some pediatric sleep specialists recommend an approach of near-constant reassurance; many others favor techniques that gently encourage an anxious baby or child to become more independent. Choose a method that conforms to your own ideas about good child rearing and matches your individual child's personality.

THE CONSTANT-REASSURANCE APPROACH

The rationale behind the constant-reassurance approach is that if you make yourself 100 percent available to your child temporarily, he'll soon come to understand that he can count on your protective presence and his separation anxiety will dissipate. Dr. Ferber elaborates: "Begin by bedding down for the night on a couch or mattress on the floor near his crib for a week or so—because your presence in your child's bedroom will reassure him. Each time he wakes up, he looks around, sees you there, and goes back to sleep without a fuss. His nighttime awakenings will soon cease." This approach may work best with a child who has customarily insisted on being held or rocked at bedtime and when he awakens during the night. "Often, he wants you to hold him not for the touching, but because he can know where you are without having to open his eyes," Dr. Ferber explains. Once he feels reassured of your availability, he'll no longer demand to be held, and once his separation anxiety has eased, you'll no longer need to sleep in his room.

INDEPENDENCE TRAINING

Other experts caution against making yourself constantly available to your anxious child. "If you try to ease your child's fears by not leaving her at all, she is denied the opportunity to learn that when her parents leave, they always come back," says Dr. Schaefer. "A child needs to learn how to be apart from her parents. Giving into her fears simply reinforces her belief that she cannot function unless attached to you." Combine the suggestions below to suit your own parenting style.

- Reassure, but don't overcomfort. "If your child panics at bedtime or naptime, stay in his room as long as it takes to calm him, but don't lift him out of the crib. Keep the light off, and don't play with him or lavish attention upon him," suggests Dr. Barton D. Schmitt. If he falls asleep, great; go about your business. If he doesn't, leave his room every 15 minutes or so, and return 1 or 2 minutes later. This teaches your child that separation is tolerable because you do come back.
- Try systematic desensitization, a process by which a fearful person is slowly and gradually introduced to the feared circumstances until she feels comfortable and unthreatened. "For a child in the throes of separation anxiety, that means gradually putting greater and greater physical distance between you and the child, until she no longer needs your pres-

ence in order to fall asleep," says Dr. Schaefer. For example, if she now sleeps in your bed, have her sleep instead on a mattress next to your bed. If she's used to snoozing on the sofa while you sit there watching TV, make up a bed of blankets for her on the floor across the room. If you usually lie next to her in her bed, sit in a chair instead. If you've been sitting next to her bed, now stand in the doorway. Do this until your child falls asleep under the new circumstances for several consecutive nights. Then continue the process, so that you slowly move farther and farther away—outside the door, down the hall, down the stairs.

· Stay in touch even when you're out of sight. If your child's separation anxiety is mild, simple tactics such as installing a night light and keeping his bedroom door open so he can hear you may be enough to put him at ease. Or he may be content if you stay on the second floor, if that's where his room is. By the time he's 1½ to 2 years old, you might suggest that he lie in bed and listen quietly for the sounds you make as you wash the dinner dishes, let the cat out, brush your teeth. If he calls out to you, don't go into his room; just call back, "I'm right here. Everything's fine."

❋

Keeping Your Emotions in Check When You're Awakened One Too Many Times

It's hard to hang onto your temper when you've been awakened for the third time in a single night by your child's piercing screams or piteous wails. "When frustrated, exhausted, and sleep deprived, even the most patient and loving parents can be overwhelmed with anger and resentment," notes Ronald E. Dahl, M.D., director of the Child and Adolescent Sleep Laboratory at the Western Psychiatric Institute and Clinic in Pittsburgh.

Try to remember that your child's behavior, though aggravating, is normal; he's reacting to stresses that are natural at his age. "Disciplinary tactics cannot stop the cries of a child truly panicked by fear," says Dr. Schaefer. "He's not being manipulative, he's crying for help." If you lose your temper, your frightened child feels even less safe, because he senses that his parent is not in control. What's more, the angrier you get, the more emotionally aroused your child gets—and the more impossible it becomes for him to fall asleep.

"But it's not enough to say to parents, 'Don't get mad,'" admits Dr. Dahl. "You will feel angry, so you need some emotional support." Find a sympathetic friend to listen while you vent your feelings. Or recruit a relative to stay overnight so you can get away for a break. A single night of uninterrupted sleep can go a long way toward replenishing reserves of parental patience and tolerance.

HELPING A CHILD HANDLE HER FEARS AND PHOBIAS

AGE FLAG: 2 TO 5 YEARS

Three-year-old Amelia lies in her bed. From the bunk above comes the sound of her big sister Alana's slow, steady breathing. But Amelia is too afraid to sleep. What if it comes again tonight, as soon as she closes her eyes? She glances fearfully at the bedroom wall. Dark, creepy, and coming toward her—there it is! "Mom, Mom, it's the shadow!" she wails.

Like a million mothers before her, Sandy Dotson rushes to comfort her frightened child. "Nothing's going to hurt you, honey," she croons. "Look, it's just the shadow of the tree outside your window." But Amelia, unconvinced, does not stop crying until her mother turns on the bedside lamp, banishing the fearsome darkness and its shadowy companions.

Nighttime fears are caused in part by a young child's inability to establish a secure boundary between reality and fantasy. A preschooler can easily imagine herself to be a superhero or princess or fairy—and can all too easily imagine the supervillains, dragons, and witches that might threaten her. During the day, she may swagger and brag, but don't expect that bravado to last long past sunset. "Kids, like adults, can often put fears out of their minds when they're playing and engaged during the day. But when they lie awake alone at night, those anxieties loom much larger," says Dr. Dahl.

❋

Kids' Most Common Nighttime Fears

Age 1 and up:	Darkness, shadows (affects 75 percent of kids by age 4); loud sounds like thunder, sirens
Age 2 and up:	Household sounds like flushing toilet, hissing radiator; imagined animals in room, such as wolves, bears, bugs

Age 3 and up:	Monsters, ghosts, ghouls; creatures that hide under beds, in closets and attics; losing bladder control during the night
Age 4 and up:	Strangers, kidnappers, robbers
Age 5 and up:	Death, injury, illness

Anything a child finds threatening can interfere with sleep. Sleep is a process of turning off our vigilance system, of relinquishing our ability to be aware of and respond to the environment. In order to fall asleep, a person must feel secure, protected, and calm. That's why it's impossible for a child to sleep when he feels afraid: his adrenaline is flowing, his mind is alert, his breathing is rapid, his eyes are open, and all his fight-or-flight mechanisms are ready for action.

Naturally, much sleep time is lost under such circumstances. "A fearful child requires almost four times longer to fall asleep than a nonfearful child, over an hour as compared with about 20 minutes," notes Dr. Schaefer. A frightened youngster also may insist on sleeping in a brightly lit room, which predisposes him to sleep lightly and thus deprives him of the deep sleep stages he needs each night.

Sometimes a child's phobias can be traced to a specific real-life event such as being menaced by a dog or accidentally locked in a dark basement. The near-universal fear of monsters may be traceable to the fact that, from the perspective of a small child, most adults and animals look huge and out of proportion. An upsurge in fears may be linked to a significant change in a youngster's life, such as starting school or moving to a new home, or to stresses imposed by parents, like overzealous toilet training or unrealistic expectations of achievement.

Often fears are generated by watching a frightening TV program or movie; even shows designed for children may be disturbing to some youngsters, as Clare Gunther learned when her daughter misinterpreted Peter Pan's character as a child-snatcher. Phobias may spring up after a child hears an upsetting story (fairy tales like "Hansel and Gretel" and nursery rhymes like "Humpty Dumpty," for instance), or learns of a violent news event. And sometimes there is no particular provocation; the child may simply realize at some point that there are scary things in the world.

Keeping the Boogie Man at Bay: How to Calm a Frightened Child

First, let's discuss what *not* to do to calm a frightened child. Never ridicule a child or scoff that her fears are nonsense. This only worsens the problem by undermining the child's self-confidence. Neither is it effective to ignore the problem. Although the object of your child's fear may not be real, the fear itself most certainly is. No matter how kind your tone of voice, telling a child that "there's nothing to be afraid of" serves only to deny the youngster's feelings and cut off conversation; it does not guide the child in dealing with her fears.

But also beware of paying too much attention to your child's fears. Being overprotective can backfire by reinforcing her frightened behavior. Because she loves getting that extra attention from Mom and Dad,

she has no motivation to overcome her fear, so don't
let an episode of night fright turn into an extension of
playtime. Instead, reward desirable behavior by prais-
ing her when she does act bravely and stays quietly in
her bed.

AGE FLAG: 1 TO 2 YEARS

If possible, help the child name her specific fear.
This may make it easier to come up with a plan to
overcome it, but if your youngster is too young to tell
you exactly what she's afraid of, don't worry. Often,
the approach will be quite similar no matter what the
child is frightened of.

How to Help Your Child Become Less Fearful

If you are calm and reassuring, you can help your child
conquer her nighttime fears.

- *Show that you are not afraid.* "A parent's facial expression and tone of voice are important cues to a
  child about whether a situation is safe. Even toddlers
  can read these cues," says Dr. Dahl. "If you act nervous, perhaps because you are concerned that your
  child's fears are a symptom of some terrible psychological trouble, this worsens the problem." Instead,
  try to project an air of calmness, strength, and confidence.
- *Avoid validating your child's fears.* Many well-
  intended attempts at providing comfort backfire because they convey the message that a child's fears
  are justified. Saying "I won't let the monsters hurt
  you" only reinforces her belief that monsters really

do exist. Turning on the bedroom light when you respond to her nighttime cries further convinces her that light is a necessary source of comfort. Letting her stay up late with you or climb into your bed validates her impression that she is not safe alone in her own room. "When your child is afraid," Dr. Schaefer suggests, "tell her, 'I'll always be nearby to comfort you when you're frightened, and I'll help you face the pretend things you're afraid of so you can go to sleep without being scared.'"

On the other hand, if the objects or events your child fears are real potential threats, acknowledge that fact and then help the child list the protective measures you've taken. Is she afraid of robbers? Show her the locks on your doors, and explain how your security system works. Is she fearful about being kidnapped? Review with her the rules against talking to or riding with strangers; teach her to recite her address and to dial her home phone number.

- *Demystify the feared objects.* Take your child outside on a warm, starry night and help her appreciate the splendor of the dark night sky. Turn on a faucet to demonstrate that those weird gurgling noises are made by the water flowing through the pipes. Transform shadows from frightening to fun by showing her how to use her hands to make shadow puppets against the wall.

- *Have your child use his imaginative skills to tame or vanquish the objects of his terror.* This helps him cope with and overcome his fears, rather than be victimized by them. For example, suggest that he think about his favorite superhero. Then he can imagine himself and the superhero together taming the wolves or tossing the robbers in jail. (Resist the temptation to put yourself in the role of hero; unless your child imagines himself taking an active part in vanquishing his foes, this exercise does not help him gain a sense of mastery over his fears.)

If your child enjoys art, he may prefer to draw a picture or make clay models of the creatures he fears. He can then tear them up or squash them as a means of ridding himself of the beasts. Or he might use his artwork to illustrate stories he makes up in which the fearsome creatures turn out to be friendly and good-hearted.

Props are effective imagination aids, too. Perhaps he can use the vacuum cleaner to vacuum up the ghosts, turn the monsters into paper airplanes and sail them out the window, or harness the "dragon" (a broomstick, a rocking horse) and ride it around the house. Do keep any such monster-mashers within reason, however. One psychologist tells of a parent who offered a child a machete with which to fend off monsters—obviously an incredibly foolhardy and dangerous thing to do.

• *Desensitize your child.* This fear-reduction procedure, as described in the section on separation anxiety above, also works well for overcoming many nighttime fears. In fact, an Australian study concluded that this technique was among the most effective and most readily accepted by children and parents alike. For example, suppose your child is afraid to be alone in bed during a thunderstorm. You might first increase her sense of familiarity and understanding by reading storybooks about thunderstorms. Next, have her sit with you and look out the window at a storm. For step three, encourage her to stay in her bed during a storm while you sit next to her in a chair. Progress to having her stay in bed while you stand in her doorway to reassure her. Then move into the next room, leaving her door open. By taking each step slowly and letting her become accustomed to it gradually, she soon should be able to weather the storm alone.

Desensitization works especially well with children who are afraid of the dark, Dr. Schaefer reports. First, install a rheostat dimmer switch (available at hardware stores) on your child's bedroom light. At bedtime let him put the dimmer on any setting he wants, even the brightest. Tell him that when he sleeps through the night at this setting without crying out, he gets a prize in the morning. If he does call out, offer comfort but no prize. Leave the light at that setting until he sleeps through three nights without obvious signs of fear. Then turn the dimmer down one notch and start over again, rewarding successful nights with a small prize. Your child will gradually adapt to an ever-darkening room, and within a month should be comfortable sleeping with only a night light.

- *Use daytime games that can motivate kids to face fears.* If your child is afraid of the dark, try this variation on hide-and-seek: hide a toy in her room, turn out the light, and encourage her to go with you to hunt for the toy. Or play follow-the-leader, leading her briefly into darkened rooms. If she's old enough to count, hold hands and go together into a dark room, then race to turn the light back on; each time you play, count to a higher number.

- *Limit your child's exposure to fear triggers.* This doesn't mean letting your child avoid all situations in which he might feel afraid. It means taking care not to expose him unnecessarily to objects or experiences that might create new fears. For instance, monitor what he watches on television or videotape. While he may not appear to be frightened during a show, scary images can creep into his mind when he's alone in bed, making it difficult for him to doze off. Do not discuss horrific news events when he's within earshot. Obviously, there are times when you'll need to talk with him about upsetting subjects, such as when a relative dies. But be careful never to equate death with sleep; otherwise, he may believe that he, too, might fall asleep one night and never wake up.

And whatever happens, try to be patient. "The first few times our daughter screamed about Peter Pan coming to take her away forever, we felt really sorry for her. But by the tenth time, my husband was only half joking when he said that wouldn't be such a bad thing," confesses Clare Gunther. Take comfort in the fact that most kids do outgrow their nighttime fears, typically by age 6 or 7.

NIGHTMARE LAND

AGE FLAG: 3 TO 6 YEARS

Kelly, age 6, dreams of being pulled through the telephone wires into an endless black void. Tammy, 5, dreams that she's in Oz, and the Scarecrow and Tin Man are chasing her around a baseball field. Three-year-old Alex dreams about being bitten by his mother's toy poodle, who has grown to the size of a house.

Look inside the dreams of any child, and you're almost guaranteed to find an occasional nightmare. Nightmares occur sporadically in virtually all children, beginning around age 6 months. "They are most common between the ages of 3 and 6, perhaps because children have an active fantasy life during this stage of development," notes Alexander K. C. Leung, M.D., clinical associate professor of pediatrics at the University of Calgary in Alberta, Canada.

Another reason youngster have more nightmares than adults—up to 10 times more, according to studies—is that children spend a greater proportion of their sleep time in REM sleep, the stage during which dreaming takes place. Most nightmares occur during the second half of the night, when REM sleep is more prevalent.

While frequent or recurring bad dreams are sometimes stress related, most nightmares have no deep-seated psychological origin and are not a cause for concern. In fact, nightmares may serve a useful teaching function. "Children often have dreams about falling, being hit by a car, or being chased by an animal—all real dangers for kids," theorizes nightmare researcher Joseph Neidhardt, M.D. "Frightening dreams may help children understand and remember the importance of avoiding such dangers."

Most nightmares are caused by, and reflect, emotional conflicts that take place during the day. Of course, any major trauma like a serious illness or accident, abuse, or a divorce or death in the family can lead to nightmares. But all types of minor conflicts can trigger bad dreams, too. "The conflict might be internal, like a 2-year-old's new sense of embarrassment related to toilet training, or a 3-year-old's sudden jealousy of a new sibling," explains Dr. Schaefer. "Or it might be external, like a neighborhood bully or an insensitive teacher." Even an infant experiences more conflict than his parents may realize, as he struggles to make sense of the bewildering array of new faces, unfamiliar events, and incomprehensible rules that confront him each day. Nightmares also may spring from a child's phobias, or vice versa; Anne Gunther's frightening dreams about Peter Pan fueled bedtime fears of him as well.

Bad dreams are more common among children with certain personality traits, such as those who bottle up their feelings, have trouble adjusting to new situations, or are especially sensitive or imaginative. They also may be triggered by a high fever, and by certain medications. Some drugs increase REM sleep, which means the child spends more sleep time in "nightmare territory." Other medications suppress REM initially, but when the drug is discontinued, the resulting rebound effect increases REM and thus also increases the likelihood of nightmares.

Whatever the source, "childhood nightmares almost always involve a specific danger to the child, such as being chased, teased, scolded, beaten, robbed, or killed," says Dr. Leung. "And they often include monsters, ghosts, devils, fierce animals, robbers, or other bad individuals." No wonder our kids wake up screaming!

How to Dispel the Terror of a Nightmare

Upon awakening from a nightmare, a child may have a feeling of suffocation and helplessness; she may feel intensely anxious, and her heart may be pounding rapidly. But unsettling as it is to see your child so frightened, it's important that you not overreact. Why? First, seeing you get upset only makes your child feel more terrified and helpless. Second, the youngster may come to feel she must protect you by concealing her nightmares, and her fears will grow. And third, she may learn that complaining about nightmares can be very rewarding in terms of the parental attention it earns her.

Instead, strive to be calm and soothing as you assure your child that she is safe and all is well. "Your child picks up on your emotional tone, or 'affect,' and soon will start to feel as though everything is all right," Dr. Neidhardt explains. You might try for some variation on this theme:

CHILD: A horrible hairy beast with huge claws was chasing me all over the backyard!

PARENT: It was a dream, honey—a picture you see in your head when you're asleep. You're awake now, so the dream is over.

CHILD: But it was trying to eat me!

PARENT: That must have been very scary. Here, let me hug you tighter. That dream is over, and it won't come back. No bad thing will happen to you.

CHILD: I want to get into your bed.

PARENT: I'll sit here next to your bed and hold your hand.

CHILD: Well, okay . . . but shut the window so the beast can't get in.

PARENT: All right. We'll shut the window to help you feel brave and ready to go back to sleep. Now give me a kiss, and close your eyes. I'll sing your bedtime song again if you like.

In this way, you accomplish several things. You remind your child that the object of her fear is not real—not to dismiss her anxiety, but to help her realize that the episode is over. You encourage her to cope with her fear by staying in her own room, rather than convey that she is incapable of protecting herself; yet with your presence, you offer the support she needs. By going along with her suggestion to shut the window, you allow her to regain a sense of control over the situation. And by repeating her favorite lullaby or some other part of her regular bedtime routine, you reestablish a sense of normalcy and security, a necessary prelude to falling back to sleep.

Resist the temptation to play detective in the middle of the night by asking lots of questions and analyzing the content of the nightmare; this could heighten the child's anxiety. The following day, however, it's wise to encourage your youngster to talk about his nightmare if he wants to. If you ignore his attempts to discuss it, he may come to feel that dreams are evil or taboo. Reassure him that many children have similar dreams, and that a nightmare is a normal, healthy way for a person to let go of something that's troubling him.

℞ *for Frequent or Recurring Nightmares*

"If your child has nightmares three to five times a week for more than a month, or frequently experiences frightening dreams with a recurrent theme, this may be a warning signal that she's struggling to deal with a specific daytime problem," explains Dr. Schaefer. In this case, use the content of the dreams to help you identify the difficulty. Dr. Neidhardt adds, "Often it's hard for parents to be objective about this, so get input from your child's daycare providers, teachers, or playmates' parents. They may give you a clue you had overlooked." Once you identify the underlying problem and take steps to solve it, the nightmares should end.

Experts also suggest several ways to defuse the power of a recurrent nightmare. Try the one that seems right for your child.

AGE FLAG: 3 YEARS AND UP

• Use storytelling skills to create a new, happier version of the dream. First, have your child describe the nightmare as it occurred, in present tense. Then have him repeat the narrative, changing the story in any way that makes him feel more comfortable. He might retell the story featuring a friendly collie instead of a frightening wolf, for example. Or he might alter the ending; instead of chasing the child and trying to eat him, the monster might simply say, "Tag—you're it!", and the story ends with a friendly game. "This is most effective if the child can come up with the new version himself," says Dr. Neidhardt. "But if he

cannot, you create a new ending and tell it to him."
This is appropriate for children between 1 and 3
years old.

Some experts suggest that the new version end
with the child destroying the monster, but others feel
it's better for the child to tame or befriend the creature that had frightened him. Dr. Neidhardt explains,
"We all need to learn to live with the monsters within
us if we are to control them."

AGE FLAG: 4 YEARS AND UP

• Art can also provide a release. First, ask your child
to draw a picture of his dream. Then encourage him
to add details that make the scene less threatening—
perhaps a police officer to arrest the evildoer, or a
baby ghost to show that the big ghost is actually a
gentle, loving mother.

Another approach is to draw the dream as it occurred, then destroy that drawing. Dr. Neidhardt describes one patient, a little girl who had been
molested, who suffered from recurrent nightmares
about a monster coming into her bedroom. After
sketching the dream, she crumpled up the paper and
threw it in the wastebasket. "All gone," she said—
and the nightmares stopped.

What if the bad dreams continue despite these efforts? "If nightmares occur at least 2 nights per week
and persist for more than 6 months, or if they are
frequent in children over 6 years of age, I'd recommend a comprehensive psychological evaluation of the
child and family," advises Dr. Leung. Seek help sooner

if nightmares are very intense, the child's daytime behavior is affected, or the problem is causing tension in the family. Your pediatrician can recommend an appropriate mental health professional.

Nightmare Prevention Tips

* Treat a toddler as if he were a bit younger than he really is so that he can meet all demands with ease. If the nightmares occur during the toilet-training period, relax the pressure to use the potty and give him more opportunities to be messy through finger-painting, mud pie making, or playing with his food.
* Encourage your child to talk freely about how she feels. But enter into these heart-to-hearts during the day, not when tucking the child into bed at night. If she goes to sleep while mulling over her problems, she's more likely to have a nightmare.
* Read storybooks to him that deal with the topics of sleep and dreams, so he better understands that everyone has dreams and that a dream cannot harm him. Preview each book yourself, to make sure the story won't be frightening to him.
* Do not let your child watch television right before bed. And restrict her viewing at all times to educational or nature shows geared to her age level. Prohibit violent shows of any kind, even cartoons.

UNDERSTANDING NIGHT TERRORS

Vera Siefert could scarcely believe what was happening. Her 4-year-old daughter, Allison, was tearing madly around the room at midnight, flailing her arms and screeching about sand creatures covering her bed. Her eyes were wide open but unfocused, and she seemed not to recognize her own mother. In fact, when Vera tried to comfort her, the child became even more agitated, pushing her mother away and screaming, "Now they're on you; they're on you, too!"

Allison was experiencing a night terror (sometimes called a sleep terror), a phenomenon that can leave parents bewildered and deeply disturbed. An episode typically begins with a piercing scream, then confused thrashing and squirming. The child may leap out of bed and run around in a panic, his eyes bulging open but glassy; often he'll hallucinate. He may mumble or cry out incoherently, or may yell, "It's going to get me!," as if in fear of attack. He shows physical signs of intense distress, such as a pounding heart, profuse sweating, and dilated pupils. He may not be aware of anyone else in the room, and if you try to soothe him, he's likely to strike out at you or react with increased horror as if you were a demon from hell.

The episode is likely to last from 10 to 30 minutes. When it's over, the child usually collapses into sleep with no memory of what happened. That's because throughout it all, he has been asleep.

Here's what happens. When a person reaches the end of a very deep sleep cycle, her brain signals that it is time to come up to a REM cycle or a brief awakening. But sometimes in children, one part of the brain wakes up while another part stays in deep sleep. The result is a night terror.

Why are children more susceptible to such episodes than adults? It's most likely associated with the relative immaturity of a child's central nervous system. Because children sleep more soundly than do adults, it is harder for them to reach REM sleep. As for why children shriek and cry during the episode, it may be that the physical symptoms of a night terror—rapid heartbeat, sweating—are associated with fear in the brain, so although there has been no real input of fear, the output is an expression of terror.

Night terrors typically occur within 1 to 3 hours after the child falls asleep, at the end of the first or second deep sleep cycle of the night. Infrequently, it may recur 3 to 4 hours later. Some youngsters experience only one night terror in the course of childhood; for others, episodes occur intermittently, perhaps one every few weeks or months for several years; occasionally, a child has one almost every night.

Up to 6 percent of children experience night terrors, with boys more often affected than girls. Episodes are most common in children 3 to 6 years old, although cases have been reported in babies as young as 6 months. Rarely, the problem may persist into the teen years. One study found that, when a child's first night terror occurred past the age of 3½, the frequency and duration of subsequent episodes were more severe than among children whose night terrors began at a younger age.

Experts generally agree that night terrors are not caused by psychological trauma. "Children experiencing night terrors are consistently found to be perfectly normal," Dr. Schaefer says. Heredity, however, does play a large part: 80 to 90 percent of children who experience night terrors have a close relative who has also encountered the problem.

Will Dobin (not his real name), can appreciate that fact: "I had night terrors as a kid, and so did my wife's younger brother. Now we're going through it with our two daughters, ages 5 and 3—and we're waiting to see if our 1-year-old son will become a 'night terrorist,' too."

Fatigue is another important element in the equation. Anything that makes a child overly tired, such as being up very late or having disturbed sleep or an erratic schedule, causes a physiological response characterized by more and deeper sleep—and this, in turn, increases the likelihood of a night terror. Episodes are especially common in children who have recently given up a nap, had a change in sleep schedule, have inconsistent sleep schedules, or just don't get as much sleep as they need.

Physical factors come into play as well. "High fevers are known to upset sleep cycles and bring on episodes of night terrors. So can pain from ear infections, surgery, or any other physical ailment," notes Dr. Schaefer. My own son, Jack, then 23 months old, had his first night terror during a long drive home from a weekend visit to Maryland—6 days after undergoing surgery to correct a double hernia.

❋

How to Tell If It's a Night Terror or a Nightmare

Night Terror	Nightmare
Occurs within 1 to 3 hours of bedtime	Occurs in second half of night
Occurs during non-REM sleep	Occurs during REM sleep

Night Terror	*Nightmare*
Not associated with dreaming	Is a frightening dream
Child remains asleep throughout	Child awakens at end of dream
During episode, child screams, thrashes; calms when terror ends	During dream, child lies quietly in bed; cries upon awakening
Child rejects attempts to comfort	Child welcomes comfort
Child has no memory of episode	Child recalls details of dream
Child returns to sleep easily	Child may be afraid to sleep

Responding to a Night Terror

Your initial reaction to the sight of your little boy or girl going berserk may be to freak out yourself. "We were terrified the first time it happened with Katie," recalls Will Dobin's wife, Diane. "There was our angelic 18-month-old screaming her head off. We thought there was something gravely wrong with her, or that we had done something terrible to cause this." Try to get a grip on yourself. Yelling at the child, bursting into tears, or calling frantically to your spouse won't help.

Even the hugging and holding that served you well when your child had a bad dream only make matters worse now. He may stiffen and push you away, or run in fear as if you were his attacker. And the more you try to comfort him, the louder he may scream. "That's because further stimulation can intensify the child's agitation, prolonging the episode," says Dr. Deborah Madansky. What's more, with all his thrashing, you may be unable to hold onto him without dropping him.

Neither is it helpful to take him into your own bed, adds Dr. Schaefer. "This does not reduce the frequency or intensity of night terrors, and can lead to other bad sleep habits." Nor should you try to awaken the child by shaking or shouting at her. In fact, if she does wake up, she may feel even more terrified and confused; children who awake from a night terror sometimes report a nameless feeling of dread and a sense of suffocation. "This probably occurs because physiologically, the child is still in a state of terror—his heart is racing, he's sweating, his mouth is dry. Once awake, he becomes consciously aware of these sensations, and that makes him even more frightened," Dr. Neidhardt explains.

So what *should* you do? Just stay with her. Diane Dobin says, "We learned to leave Katie in her crib, though it was the hardest thing just to stand by doing nothing while our tiny child was in the throes of this fit." Actually, you're not doing nothing. You're keeping her safe by preventing her from running into a wall, breaking a window, or falling down the stairs. And when the episode is finally over, you can settle her back into bed.

The following day, your child probably won't recall the incident at all. There's no need to describe the scene in graphic detail, or interrogate him about it. Discourage siblings from teasing the child about his nighttime screaming and crying, as this can be quite embarrassing. But do discuss the situation with your babysitter, explaining what a night terror is and how it should (and shouldn't) be handled in your absence.

In most cases, night terrors taper off and eventually disappear as the child's nervous system matures, but you may want to seek professional help if episodes are occurring almost nightly, or if the problem persists past age 11. Psychotherapy, medication, or hypnosis can often solve the problem.

Prevention Tactics for Night Terrors

There are several steps you can take to prevent night terrors:

• Don't let your child become overtired. "Very tired children spend more time in deep sleep states. Extending the time spent in night-terror territory increases their likelihood," cautions Dr. Schaefer. So stick to a regular bedtime schedule, even during vacations and holidays, and enforce daytime naps or rest periods.

• Keep the pre-bedtime hour from becoming too rambunctious. Some parents report an increase in episodes when the kids have had an evening pillow fight or tickle session with Dad.

• Make bedtime light and happy. Though night terrors are generally considered a physiological phenomenon, it doesn't hurt to consider psychological factors as well. Says Dr. Dahl, "If your child tends to ruminate on his problems as he lies in bed, redirect his thoughts toward happier things. Perhaps he can name all the people who love him, or think of three good things that happened that day, or plan a fun outing for tomorrow."

• For frequent night terrors, try prompted awakenings. "The theory is that night terrors are caused by a faulty deep sleep phase; when that disturbed pattern is interrupted, the child reverts to a normal sleep pattern," explains Dr. Schaefer. First, keep a sleep diary for 1 or 2 weeks, noting how many minutes elapse from the time your child falls asleep until the onset of the night terror. Then, awaken the child 15 minutes before the time the terror typically begins. Keep him fully awake and out of bed for 5 minutes, then settle him back to sleep. Carry out these prompted awakenings for 7 consecutive nights, then stop. If the terrors return, repeat the 7-night program. Reported success rate of this technique is an impressive 90 percent. Diane Dobin is a believer: "It worked for our younger daughter, Rebecca. In the 9 months since we did this, she's had scarcely any night terrors. What a relief!"

---------------- ✳ ----------------

Storybooks to Banish Bad Dreams and Night Frights

Reading a relevant story with your child can show him that he's not alone with his fears, encourage him to talk about the things that frighten him, give you both some good ideas for overcoming the problem, and introduce a welcome bit of levity to the situation. Here are some titles to look for:

Alex Fitzgerald's Cure for Nightmares, by Kathleen Krull

Bedtime for Frances, by Russell Hoban

Ben's Dream, by Chris van Allsberg

Harry and the Terrible Whatzit, by Dick Gackenbach

I Had a Bad Dream: A Book About Nightmares, by Linda Hayward

In the Night Kitchen, by Maurice Sendak

Jessica and the Wolf, by Ted Lobby

My Mama Says There Aren't Any Zombies, Ghosts or Vampires, by Judith Viorst

Storm in the Night, by Mary Stolz

The Berenstain Bears and the Bad Dream, by Stan and Jan Berenstain

The Monster at the End of the Book, by Jon Stone

The Monster Is Coming, by Michaela Morgan and Sue Porter

There's a Nightmare in My Closet, by Mercer Mayer

What's Under My Bed?, by James Stevenson

Where the Wild Things Are, by Maurice Sendak

Who's Afraid of the Dark?, by Crosby Bonsall

✳

✺ FIVE

Where Should Your Child Sleep?

When you were pregnant, it probably seemed like a simple decision. You'd convert the guest room to a nursery, buy a beautiful new crib, perhaps borrow that heirloom bassinet from your sister. And then you'd be ready to welcome this darling new creature into your heart and your home.

But in truth, it doesn't always work out that way. You lay your newborn babe in her crib, but she cries—and the bed seems so vast compared to her tiny form. So you put her in the bassinet next to the crib, hoping she'll find it cozier, yet again she screams in protest. Then you wheel the bassinet into your bedroom, thinking that if she can see you lying next to her, she'll settle down. She doesn't. So you scoop her up and lay her in your bed, sandwiched between your husband's body and your own. Maybe she falls asleep, maybe she doesn't. Maybe you fall asleep, maybe you don't. Either way, you wonder: am I doing the right thing?

Or maybe your child's already a bit older. He's begun to climb out of his crib and you're afraid he'll fall. Is it time for a big-boy bed? Will he balk at such a change? Or will he think this gives him license to run unrestrained through the house at night?

Figuring out the best place for your child to sleep can be a tricky business. Trickier still, oftentimes, is convincing your child to cooperate. This chapter presents the pros and cons of various sleeping arrangements, and suggests ways that you can change your current situation if it's proving problematic.

INFANTS ONLY: THE BEST PLACE FOR A SLUMBERING NEWBORN

Many parents opt for a crib, confident that those high side rails will keep their baby safe. Such confidence is well placed, provided the crib meets all current Consumer Product Safety Commission standards. (Older cribs may not.) If your tiny newborn seems lost in the vastness of the crib, make him feel more secure by swaddling him in a blanket, or by placing him in a corner of the crib with his head just touching a bumper pad.

Some newborns seem to feel more at ease with the snugger fit a bassinet provides. This is also a fine option for the first several months, provided the bassinet checks out for safety. Parents may appreciate the bassinet's mobility, wheeling the baby to any convenient spot in the house during her naps, and then into their own room at bedtime so she'll be handy for nighttime feedings.

This strategy can backfire, however, if it is allowed to go on too long. "I have 14 children," says veteran mom Rose Mary Wood. "All my babies slept in a bassinet next to my bed for the first 6 weeks or so, then moved into a bedroom with one of their siblings. But by the time we had Michaela, our youngest, the house was so full that there simply was no other bedroom to put her in. She's 8 months old now, and still sleeps in the crib next to me. Wouldn't you know, she's the only one of all my kids to have any sleep problems? She still wakes up twice a night to eat, and I go ahead and feed her because I can't bear to hear her cry while I'm lying just a few feet away."

If you do opt for a bassinet, it's probably wise to move it into the child's own room by the time she's 4 to 6 weeks old. Retire the bassinet altogether no later than the baby's 3-month birthday. By that time, she'll have grown so much that the bassinet will have become too cramped for comfort.

Some parents let their baby snooze in an infant seat during the day, so they can move the napping baby with them from room to room. "Provided she sleeps well at night, there's no reason to restrict your baby's napping to the crib," says Dr. Richard Ferber. "But if she has any nighttime sleep problems, you're better off using her crib consistently during the day and night, so she gets used to sleeping there."

When a baby suffers from gastroesophageal reflux (very frequent spitting up due to an abnormality of the esophagus), the traditional advice has been to place him in his infant seat after every meal, whether he's awake or asleep. The theory is that when he's in a semiupright position, gravity will help the food stay down in his stomach. However, recent studies indicate that the upright position may actually worsen reflux, because it places added pressure on the abdomen. If your baby suffers from reflux, ask your pediatrician whether sleeping in an infant seat is recommended or not.

On His Stomach or on His Back?

For decades, parents were advised to lay an infant down on her stomach, to reduce the risk that the child would choke if she happened to vomit in her sleep. Recently, though, the American Academy of Pediatrics reversed its opinion on this, and now recommends that a baby sleep on her back or side. The reason: new studies indicate that the face-down position may double a baby's susceptibility to sudden infant death syndrome (SIDS).

AGE FLAG: NEWBORN TO 12 MONTHS

SIDS, which strikes 7,000 infants in this country each year and is the leading cause of death for infants 2 to 6 months old, is defined as the sudden death of a child under age 1 that cannot be otherwise explained. Experts theorize that, when a baby is lying face down, he may not be able to take in enough oxygen because he is "rebreathing" air from a small pocket of bedding pulled up around his nose. In effect, he suffocates. The risk is especially high when a baby is sleeping on a quilt, waterbed, or sheepskin.

There are some exceptions to the new rule. If your baby was born prematurely, vomits excessively, or has certain facial defects, your pediatrician may recommend that she sleep on her stomach, with her head carefully turned to one side.

For the majority of infants, however, the rule to remember is "back to sleep." What if your baby doesn't like to sleep on his back? "Try placing him on his side instead, using a rolled-up blanket behind his back to support him in this position," suggests Dr. Deborah Madansky. To keep him from rolling onto his tummy, arrange his lower arm at a right angle to his body. To help him associate the side-lying position with happy experiences, several times a day you might lay him on his side, then lie down next to him and talk, sing, or nurse.

AGE FLAG: 3 TO 5 MONTHS

Once your baby can roll over, you may have a harder time keeping her on her back. Try using cushioned wedges, one on either side of her body, to prevent her from rolling over. Or hang an interesting mobile above her crib, so she decides that looking up at this fascinating thing is more fun than looking down at the mattress.

THE FAMILY BED: IS IT RIGHT FOR YOU?

When it comes to kids and slumber, few issues seem to stir up as much passionate debate as the one about cosleeping—the term psychologists use to describe the practice of parents sharing sleeping space with their children. Staunch supporters believe that all children belong in their parents' beds, all night, every night, from the time they're born until they choose to leave, whether that choice is made at 10 weeks, 10 months, or 10 years of age.

Dissenters, however, claim that cosleeping causes a multitude of daytime and nighttime problems, and should be strongly discouraged. And then there are parents who position themselves in the middle of the cosleeping road, preferring not to make the family bed an every-night policy, but allowing the kids into the king-size at certain times.

Again, there's no one course that's right for every family. The cosleeping question is a highly personal one, and the way in which you answer it must reflect your values, beliefs, and parenting style. This section discusses the pros and cons of the family bed, suggests factors to consider in making your decision, and then offers practical tips for implementing whichever policy you choose—be it to invite your children into your bed or to persuade them to stay out.

The Case for Cosleeping

When parents share their bed with their children, champions of cosleeping say, a host of benefits are realized.

• A child's sense of emotional well-being is encouraged. "I believe that children who are ignored and left to cry at night may feel unimportant and unloved. So by welcoming my children into my bed, I help them feel safe and secure," says Elizabeth Pantley, a mother of three.

Some parents opt to offer that reassurance beginning right at bedtime, by letting their child fall asleep in the parents' bed and spend the whole night there. Others put their child to bed in her own room, but willingly make space for her in their bed should she cry out or come to them in the middle of the night. It's a simple and loving way, they say, to get everyone back to sleep when a toddler is terrified by a nightmare, or when a preschooler wets her own bed and asks to be warmed in yours.

· Parent–child bonding is enhanced. "Since I work full time, sleeping together gives me many more hours to spend with my infant son. It's wonderful to open my eyes and see that angelic baby face next to mine," says Lisa Sharkey Gleicher, mother of two boys.

Nor is the emotional closeness of the family bed limited to parents of infants, proponents point out. "My firstborn is 9 years old now, so I don't get to hold him in my lap much anymore. That's why I relish the chance to cuddle him whenever he decides to pop into bed with my husband and me," says Sarah Frank (not her real name), mother of four.

· For nursing mothers, cosleeping can be a convenience. "With my first baby, I'd get up at 2 A.M. to feed him, fall asleep in the chair, and almost drop him. I felt like I never got a decent night's sleep, and I was always exhausted during the day," says Lisa Gleicher. "So now my second baby sleeps with me, and I doze lying down while he nurses. I get a lot more rest than I did when my oldest was a baby, and during the day I feel alert and energized."

· Bed sharing may quiet nighttime disturbances. "William used to wake up and cry several times each night. Then once he learned to climb out of his crib, he'd walk quietly into our room and just stand there. I'd wake up from a sound sleep and find his face inches from mine, these big eyes staring down at me. It was really unnerving," says Audrey Cope, mother of one. "Finally, we just moved a foamy cushion into our room and made up a bed for William right next to our own. If he stirred at night, my husband could just lean over and pat him, and William would go right back to sleep."

• It's common practice in much of the rest of the world—and more common in this country than many people realize. "Parents and children sleeping together is the norm in most contemporary cultures, including industrialized societies like Japan," says James McKenna, Ph.D., professor of anthropology at Pomona College in Claremont, California. In fact, cosleeping was routine in America until this century. Even today studies show that more than half of families with children ages 2 to 3 sleep together at least occasionally, while more than 10 percent always share a bed.

• Cosleeping may be protective. "From an evolutionary perspective, cosleeping was beneficial—a matter of survival," says Dr. McKenna. That makes sense. Infants too young to digest mammoth meat needed around-the-clock access to Mother's breasts. In the absence of central heating, cave babies relied on Mom's body heat for warmth. Unable to run and hide, tiny tots left alone at night were easy prey for predators.

AGE FLAG: NEWBORN TO 12 MONTHS

Admittedly, protecting a child from stalking beasts is but a minor concern on Main Street, U.S.A.—but protecting a child from SIDS is a major one. While the evidence is by no means conclusive, some research suggests that cosleeping may in some cases provide an added safeguard against SIDS. Dr. McKenna explains, "Infants who sleep with a parent spend less time in the two deepest stages of sleep, and wake up more often than babies who sleep alone. This is important because all infants stop breathing briefly several times during the night, and babies who fail to come out of deep sleep and take a breath are at greater risk for SIDS."

Arguments Against Bunking with Baby

Before you let yourself be persuaded by the enthusiasm of cosleeping's supporters, consider the potential down side as well. First, the concerns about kids who cosleep:

• The sad fact is, a child can be injured or even killed while sleeping in an adult bed. The danger is greatest for infants, of course. More than 250 infants suffocated in adult beds between 1985 and 1990, either when another person rolled onto them or, more commonly, when they slipped between the mattress and wall or bed frame. Risk is highest on a very soft mattress or waterbed, or when a parent has been taking medication or drinking. Less tragic but still troublesome is the possibility that a young child might suffer a broken bone if he falls out of bed or if a sleeping adult rolls on top of him.

- Cosleeping may make sleep problems worse. A University of Massachusetts study found that toddlers who sleep with parents are up to 10 times more likely not to want to sleep alone, and are two to four times as likely to have trouble falling asleep or to wake up during the night. Why? Researchers conclude that bed sharing can provide positive reinforcement for nighttime awakenings and prevent a child from learning how to settle herself down.

- Children may become overly dependent if the family bed continues for more than a couple years. "The task of a 2- or 3-year-old is to become more autonomous. Cosleeping doesn't necessarily prevent that, but it certainly doesn't promote it," says Dr. Charles E. Schaefer. Later, a child who can't leave his parents' bed may be unable to do the things his friends do—attend sleepovers, go away to camp.

- A parents' big bed can dispel the terror of a bad dream or ease anxiety over an isolated problem with a playmate. Yet if a child needs such reassurance night after night, cosleeping provides only a temporary fix at best. "If a youngster is afraid of the dark or of being alone, and you deal with her fear by sleeping with her, you're not really solving the problem of what is causing this underlying fear," explains Dr. Schaefer. (For more information on nighttime fears, refer to Chapter Four.)

- Cosleeping may cause sexual confusion among the preschool and early school-age set. "Children this age often feel intensely infatuated with the parent of the opposite sex, and sharing a bed may be overly stimulating," says Dr. Schaefer. Resentment can be particularly strong if a boy is allowed into bed with Mom or a girl with Dad only when the other parent is traveling, and then is displaced when the parent returns. Or the child of divorced parents may resent having to move out of the bed to make room for a parent's new partner.

Another concern is that a bed-sharing child might not be able to distinguish between a family member's innocent snuggles and another person's inappropriate advances. Marla Duncan (not her real name), mother of one girl, says, "I'm afraid that if I teach my daughter it's okay to sleep with her daddy, she'll think it's also all right to lie down with a babysitter or some old man down the street."

Parents who are considering an open-bed policy should also factor in the potential problems they themselves might encounter:

- You may get less sleep—a lot less. "It's well documented that the more people there are in one bed, the less soundly parents will sleep," notes Dr. Ferber. Remember, kids tend to twist and turn and mumble and moan in their sleep, and all that commotion may keep you awake.

  Lisa Kristal-Abrams, whose son has become a permanent guest in her bed, admits, "Our 2-year-old sleeps every which way. He puts his feet in our faces and his fingers in our eyes, he grabs pillows and kicks off covers. My husband and I can't get a wink of sleep." Lisa initially liked the idea of a family bed—but the reality has left her disillusioned and desperate for shut-eye.

- Once your child gets used to sleeping with you, she

may not want to stop. It's the proverbial slippery slope: start down the cosleeping path, and soon there may be no turning back. "Chase always slept fine in his own bed, until one night when he was sick and we brought him in with us," explains Lisa. "After that, there seemed to be no way to get him out."

Even parents philosophically committed to bed sharing may eventually question their decision to let the child call the shots. One friend of a friend signed herself out of the hospital against medical advice just hours after giving birth, because the staff wouldn't let her newborn sleep with her around the clock. Now that child is 4, still sleeps all night in her parents' bed, and the mother is asking herself, "Is this going to last forever?"

Too often, it seems, the newborn who was welcomed eagerly into bed is still sandwiched between Mom and Dad, less welcome, a year later. Or a toddler whose earache needed soothing refuses to return to her room, many months after the pain has passed. Or a kid climbs into the king-size only once or twice a week, which wouldn't be so bad except that, for Pete's sake, he's 10 years old and isn't enough enough already! Sure, some children do elect privacy over day-and-night parenting, usually by age 4—but not all do. "If parents don't like the idea of sleeping with a 5-year-old, it's probably best not to start with a 5-month-old," says Dr. Schaefer.

· Cosleeping complicates your sex life. No, you can't just wait for the child to fall asleep. "Having sex while a child's in the room is not wise; she may awaken and misinterpret the parents' actions as violent or hurtful," explains Dr. Ferber. While some family-bed enthusiasts claim an off-limits bedroom is an incentive to seek romance elsewhere in the house, other couples are turned off by the idea of quickies in the kitchen. "Finding time for sex is hard enough without having to find a place, too," says my sister Barbara Eberlein, mother of two.

- A child who's used to sleeping with you may not be able to drop off unless you go to bed, too—at 8 o'clock in the evening—even though you might prefer to stay up till 11. Or she might refuse to stay with a sitter, because she won't be able to get to sleep in your absence. And even if you're not planning a night on the town, you probably cherish those hours between the kids' bedtime and your own. It may be the only time you have to talk to your partner uninterrupted and uncensored, to play piano or polish your nails, to curl up with a book that doesn't begin "Once upon a time . . ." Such moments replenish reserves of parental patience, and so cannot be sacrificed lightly.

- When both parents embrace the philosophy, cosleeping can bring them even closer—but if one partner resents the child's presence, problems may arise. Some parents resolve the conflict by buying a guardrail and having the family-bed enthusiast, rather than the baby, sleep in the middle. But, Dr. Schaefer cautions, "it's asking for trouble if one parent who can't sleep with the thrashing child leaves the bed to sleep elsewhere, in effect allowing the youngster to take his or her place."

To Share or Not to Share? How to Decide for Yourself

Before you make a hard-and-fast decision, tune in to your child's needs. Through trial and error, you may find that your child thrives on communal nights; or you may discover that she resists sharing sleep space. "You can have a perfectly well-nurtured child either way," says Dr. Schaefer. "Just be sure, if you sleep apart, that the child gets plenty of attention and affection during the day. If you bunk down together, provide him with other opportunities for privacy."

Next, examine your own motives. If you cosleep because you believe it enhances family closeness, that's fine. But it should not be done to alleviate adult anxiety or loneliness, or as an excuse for avoiding intimacy with your partner.

Finding a Comfortable Middle Ground

Cosleeping doesn't have to be an all-or-nothing arrangement. Here are some alternatives:

* Rather than bring the baby into your bed, put her bassinet in your room.
* If sharing sleep space with your preschooler is like bunking with a wriggling eel, have him sleep on a cot or mattress next to your bed instead.
* Let your little one into your bed on Friday and Saturday nights only. Both parents and child have the option of sleeping in if you need to.
* Tell your youngster he's welcome in your bed every day—provided he waits until the sun comes up to join

you. If he arrives too early on any given morning, escort him back to his own bed immediately.

- If you have several children, create a sibling sleeping room, as Elizabeth Pantley did. "Our three children slept with us when they were babies. Then we decided to let them all share one king-size mattress in another room. I lie down with the kids at bedtime each night for a while, and then I get up and go about my evening activities. The three of them snuggle together and enjoy the comfort of each other's presence during the night."

Does your spouse agree with your stance on cosleeping? If not, resentment will surely result. For instance, if he asks, "With the kids in our bed, where will we make love?", you can't dismiss his concern. Instead, work together to come up with solutions you can both accept—making love in the guest room, on the sleeper sofa in the den, or in your own bedroom (with the door locked) while the kids watch Saturday-morning cartoons.

Consider, too, how you might handle the potential problems inherent in the arrangement you choose. If you do opt for cosleeping, for instance, be prepared to explain to your child that cuddling in bed is strictly a family thing. You might tell her that it's just like bathing: while it's okay for Mom or Dad to give her a bath, nobody else should—and in the same way, nobody else should try to coax her into bed, either.

Whatever you decide, let go of guilt. You're entitled to privacy if that's what you want, and forcing yourself to share your bed won't make kids feel secure if it makes you tense. On the other hand, if the family bed just feels right, then go for it. "Parents are in the best position to judge what their own child needs, and what they themselves feel comfortable with," says Dr. McKenna, because in the end, sleeping with your child is not a question of right or wrong. It's a matter of personal preference.

How to Convince a Cosleeper to Relocate

When the time comes to change the arrangement, here are some ways to get your child to stay in his own room:

- To make the child's room more inviting, let him help select a new bedspread, poster, or goldfish. Be sure the bedtime ritual ends with tucking the youngster into his own bed. Avoid daytime punishment that involves sending the child to his room.
- Help your youngster bond with a teddy or blanket by encouraging her to cuddle it while you hold her. Soon she'll find it comforting whether you're with her or not. Bob Michaels (not his real name), father of a 3-year-old, reports, "When my wife and I decided that Gina should go back to sleeping in her own bed, we asked our daughter if she could think of any ways to make the change easier. Gina came up with a great idea. She said that because her stuffed dinosaur Dinky had always slept with her ever since she was a baby, Dinky would be company enough for her when she moved into her own bed."
- If cold turkey seems harsh, make the switch step by

step. First have your child nap in his own bed during the day; once he's adjusted, tackle the nighttime habit. Or make the move gradually by first moving the child from your bed to a crib or cot a few feet away. Over the course of 1 or 2 weeks, ease his bed toward the door, then into the hall, and finally into his room. Make the process more fun by telling the child he's "camping out."

· Motivate a preschooler with a star chart for successful nights spent in his room. By the time you're up to 15 stars, the cosleeping habit should be broken. Or use whatever your family considers to be a reward worth working for. Jennifer Trillo, mother of three girls, says, "The first time our 4-year-old stayed in her own room all night instead of climbing into bed with us, we made a big fuss over her in the morning and told her how wonderfully she'd behaved. Then we awarded her the prize that represents, in our family, the ultimate mark of approval: cookies for breakfast."

How to Eliminate Sneaking

AGE FLAG: 2 YEARS AND UP

It's 2 A.M., you're dead tired, and your child has just sneaked silently into your room. If you're serious about putting a halt to bed sharing, your course of action is clear: you must get up and escort the child back to her room immediately. Don't yell, plead, or punish. Simply tuck her in, tell her she's safe, then leave. Do this no matter how many times she tries to climb into your bed in the middle of the night.

Suppose your savvy kid slides into your bed so

stealthily that you don't even wake up. If he manages to remain there for several hours before being discovered, he'll probably feel his efforts have been adequately rewarded even if he's eventually returned to his own room. That means you need to wake up as soon as he sneaks into your room. Try placing a bell on your doorknob to signal the child's arrival—but don't lock him out of your room; it's never safe to let a child roam through the house alone at night.

If all else fails, try "crowding" the kid, Dr. Schaefer suggests. "While pretending to be asleep, stretch your arms out over his face, roll on top of him, push him to the edge of the bed. If he falls out, don't say a word. If he climbs between you and your spouse, move toward the middle and squish him. Eventually, he'll decide his own bed is more comfortable than yours."

MAKING THE BIG MOVE FROM CRIB TO BED

AGE FLAG: 18 TO 36 MONTHS

Peter Dilsheimer, 20 months, was a man with a mission. He swung his leg over the side rail of the crib, and hoisted up his bottom until he was sitting astride the railing. He inched his way forward till he arrived at the head of the bed. Then with great derring-do, he launched himself through the air and landed atop the cable TV box, which was perched on top of a portable television, which was sitting on a small end table. The whole kit and caboodle, kid included, crashed to the floor. "I heard this terrible crash and dashed in to see what had happened," says Peter's mother, Barbara. "When I saw the wreckage, my first reaction was, thank God he's not hurt. My second one was, this crib has got to go. The very next day, we set up Peter's new twin bed."

Plan to make the switch to a regular bed as soon as your child learns to climb out of his crib when the mattress springs are at their lowest setting. Expect this to occur sometimes between the ages of 18 and 36 months, or whenever your youngster reaches about 32 inches in height. Don't delay; if the child falls while climbing out of the crib, he could be injured. Neither is it wise to attempt to reduce the risk of a fall by placing a chair next to the crib; this may just encourage more acrobatics.

I was dismayed when my twins started climbing out of their cribs many months before their second birthday—I hadn't expected this development yet, and I certainly wasn't prepared for it. I knew I needed to order beds pronto, but how would I keep my little monkeys safe until the new furniture arrived? The answer: dismantle the cribs, place the crib mattresses directly on the floor, and let the twins sleep there. Then, if they rolled off, at least they'd only fall a few inches.

If you can't bear the thought of letting your little one roam free just yet, consider buying a crib tent, a dome-shaped structure made of net that attaches over the top of the crib. The tent keeps a tot inside the crib without tying him down or making him claustrophobic. "You needn't feel guilty about 'caging' a child when you use a tent," adds Dr. Jodi Mindell. "The child has effectively been caged in her crib all along."

Suppose your child never does try to climb out of her crib? Then you can safely continue to use the crib for a while longer, until the child reaches a height of 36 inches.

If you're expecting another baby and plan to use the crib for the newborn, it's best to switch your older child to a big bed at least 3 months before your due date. "A few weeks is simply not enough time for your firstborn to stop feeling proprietary about the old crib, and the sight of a new sibling in 'her' crib can be unsettling for a youngster," explains Dr. Mindell. Your older child is still too young to sleep in a big bed? Buy her a new crib that converts to a youth bed, and move her into it well before the baby arrives. Later on, when she's ready, simply convert the new crib to a youth bed.

How to Choose a Big-Kid Bed

* If your youngster's room is large enough, consider getting a full-size double bed. The added roominess allows greater freedom of movement while sleeping, and provides more comfort for parent and child during quiet talks and bedtime reading.
* For maximum comfort and support for a growing body, invest in a quality mattress and box spring.
* To keep the child from rolling out of bed as he sleeps, use detachable safety rails.
* Bunk beds are not recommended for children under age 6. If you want bunks, buy the type that can also be configured as two separate twin beds; use them as twins now, and convert them to bunk beds a few years down the road.

Preparing a Child for the Big Move

Switching to a regular bed represents an important milestone in your child's life. You can ease the transition by scheduling the move for a time when no other major changes (toilet training, weaning, giving up the pacifier) are taking place.

You can encourage your child to feel enthusiastic about the idea of a big bed by using words like these:

PARENT: Sally, I have some exciting news. Remember how I told you a few weeks ago that I had bought a new bed for you, the kind that big kids sleep in? Well, the new bed will be delivered to our house tomorrow, so today, we can go to the store together and pick out a bedspread and some sheets to use on your new bed.

CHILD: Can I have a Little Mermaid bedspread?

PARENT: Sure, if that's what you want. Maybe we'll even find a matching Mermaid poster to hang on the wall.

CHILD: Okay. I like that.

PARENT: And then tomorrow we'll invite Grandma and Grandpa to dinner for a Big Bed Party, to celebrate.

CHILD: Can we have a cake, too? And balloons?

PARENT: Good idea. Then after dinner, we'll put on your pajamas and tuck you into your new big-girl bed for the very first time.

CHILD: Oh, that will be fun!

This parent talks about the arrival of the bed as an event her youngster can look forward to with pride. By inviting the child to help shop for the new linens and wall decorations, the parent increases her daughter's sense of control over the switch. And with the party, the move to a big bed becomes a happy celebration.

When a Child Balks at Sleeping in the New Bed

Some kids need extra coaxing before they can adapt to the change. Tactics to try:

- Go gradually. Start by putting just the mattress on the floor, and let the child sleep there. Once he's used to that, add the box spring. Finally, set up the entire bed. Or, set up the new bed near the crib; have the child take naps in the bed but use the crib at night. Once he feels ready to spend the whole night in the bed, retire the crib permanently.
- Avoid unnecessary additional changes. Place the bed in the same location where the crib had been. Cover the child with her old crib blanket, even if it's too small. Follow the same bedtime ritual as before.
- Add an element of fun. Decorate a carton and fill it with toys and books that are "just for kids who sleep in a big bed." Include a few old favorites from the crib, as well as some new items. One universal favorite: a flashlight she can play with in bed.
- Use story-telling as a nonconfrontational strategy. Pick one of your child's favorite characters—Mickey Mouse, for example—and pretend that he couldn't

stay in his new bed, either. Explain how Mickey tried Donald Duck's bed, then Goofy's bed, and finally the floor, but none were right for him. In the story, Mickey then asks your child for advice and your youngster wisely tells him that sleeping in his own bed is the solution to his problem because it's made just for him.

How to Halt Night Wanderings

AGE FLAG: 2 TO 5 YEARS

You got your kid into a big bed, but now the problem is that she won't stay there. When she said goodbye to her crib, she said goodbye, too, to the external controls that formerly kept her from jumping up and running out of her room.

For you, there may be some small consolation in knowing you're not alone: in a *Child* magazine survey, parents reported that refusing to stay in bed was one of the most common sleep problems among preschoolers. But of course, what you really want to know is how to put a stop to those night wanderings. Fortunately, you have a number of options.

Start by clearly stating the new rule. "Once our bedtime ritual is over and I've tucked you into bed, you may not leave your room." Be sure to anticipate any legitimate needs—to use the potty, have a drink of water, locate the stuffed Barney he always sleeps with—and meet them in the course of the bedtime routine. If after he's in bed, he calls out that he's thirsty or needs to go to the bathroom, tell him to take care of it himself and then to get straight back into bed.

Provide positive reinforcement for cooperative behavior—praise, a star chart, a small prize.

The problem persists? Then you need to select a strategy for enforcing the rule. Choose the one or ones below that seem best suited to your individual situation.

THE SILENT-ESCORT APPROACH

Most experts agree that the first line of defense should be to simply escort the child silently back to bed. You might remind her that she must stay in her room, but beyond that, don't say a word. Certainly do not reward her wanderings by allowing her to stay up awhile, reading an extra story, or offering additional hugs and kisses. Don't lecture or scold her, either; even negative attention may be more attractive to her than none at all. If she truly needs to use the bathroom and cannot yet manage this on her own, help her. But keep such potty trips neutral; there's no need to make them fun.

What if she leaves her room once more? Calmly and wordlessly return her to bed again—and again, and again, and again, as many times as it takes to show her that you mean business. "If after the tenth time she sneaks out of her room, you throw your hands up in despair and let her join you in front of the TV, you are asking for trouble," warns Dr. Lee J. Brooks. "The key to success is to be 100 percent consistent in returning the child to her room immediately." Do not waver; she'll eventually get the message. If she doesn't, move on to one of the methods outlined below.

THE DOOR-CLOSING METHOD

Try this with a child who continues to leave his room no matter how often you escort him back. When you tuck the child in at bedtime, warn him that if he pops up, you will have to close his bedroom door—and it will stay closed until he's back under his covers.

He'll probably get out of bed just to test you. At this point, shut the door from the outside and hold it closed for 1 minute. Then open it and restate the rule: that as long as the child stays in bed, the door stays open. If he still won't cooperate, hold the door closed for a longer period. Does he throw a tantrum? Open the door, put him back into bed, then hold the door closed again until the child stays down. "The point of this is to give the child a choice in the situation. *He* is in charge of the door, because his own behavior determines whether the door stays open or closed," explains Dr. John Herman. "Hard as it might be, try not to get mad, because that gives a child the message that he is bad. If you can control your anger, however, you'll be more effective at helping the child learn what he needs to learn."

THE BARRICADE METHOD

"While a youngster may welcome the big-kid status her new bed confers, she may also be disturbed by the expectation of self-control that accompanies it," says Dr. Ferber. The idea behind the barricade method is to replace the external controls that were lost when the crib disappeared, so that the child has help in overcoming her impulse to leave her room at night.

First, be certain the bedroom is well babyproofed. Then place a gate across the doorway to prevent the child from leaving—in effect, turning the entire room into a crib. "You do this not to punish or frighten the child, but to show her that control is there," Dr. Ferber explains. If she cries, return to the doorway briefly to reassure her that all is well, but do not take down the gate or pick up the child. If her protests continue, you can return to her doorway after increasingly lengthy intervals, to reassure her and restate the rule again. Keep such visits very brief, and do not let yourself be drawn into conversation.

Does your little acrobat figure out how to climb over the gate, as my son, Jack, did? Try using two gates, one on top of the other. Or take a tip from my neighbor, who cut his child's door in half horizontally and added some extra hinges to create a Dutch-style door that could be locked at the bottom but left open at the top.

THE LAST-RESORT, LOCKED-DOOR APPROACH

Many experts discourage parents from locking a child in his room. "It's a safety hazard. What if there was a fire? The child would be trapped," warns Dr. Mindell.

"Sleep is something a child needs, not something you impose on him as punishment," adds Dr. Brooks. "If you lock a child in, his bedroom becomes a jail. This is not at all the healthy attitude you want to instill." After trying this technique on her 2-year-old son, Charlene Barrett (not her real name) concedes that it was a disaster: "Joey went ballistic when I locked him in his room. He ripped up all his books, bent the Venetian blinds, pulled out all his dresser drawers, tossed his clothes all over the floor. By the time I unlocked the door, the place looked like a battle-field."

But some experts say that, as a last resort, door-locking has a legitimate place in parents' sleep-training manuals. "If your child learns to climb over a barri-cade, a full door may need to be kept closed until morning with a hook, piece of rope, or chain lock. While you may consider this step extreme, it can be critical for protecting children less than 5 years old who wander through the house at night without an understanding of the dangers—the stove, hot water, electricity, knives, going outdoors," asserts Dr. Barton D. Schmitt.

If you feel you have no choice but to lock the door, yet can't bear for your child to be so isolated, consider replacing her regular bedroom door with a very sturdy screen door or Plexiglas door. This way you can see in and the child can see out—but she cannot get out and go wandering.

✻ SIX

Solutions to Special Situations

It's frustrating to scrutinize a book on parenting and not find any mention of a specific, unique problem you're facing—things like backsliding after an illness, how to handle bedtime routines when you're traveling, or the sleep problems unique to siblings who share a room. Or you might suspect that your child has a sleep disorder that requires professional help. In this chapter, we'll address all these concerns, and more.

BANISHING BACKSLIDING

It's an unfortunate fact of parenting that you can never depend 100 percent on a child's sleep being problem-free. With appropriate training, she may go for weeks or even months sleeping like an angel with nary a protest or disturbance, but at some point she's bound to backslide a bit—or even a lot. There are several reasons why a return to bad sleeping habits can happen:

- *Developmental changes.* "My baby boy John had been sleeping through the night for several months. But now he's 7 months old and has just learned to crawl. I think his little body is so busy exploring the world and his little brain so excited by all his new discoveries that when he awakens at 2 A.M., he's simply too jazzed up to fall back to sleep," says Marey Oakes, a mother of three.

AGE FLAG: 5 TO 10 MONTHS

Marey's probably right. "The excitement and frustration of learning new skills such as sitting, creeping, and crawling carry over into the night. A baby's naps may be disrupted, too, as she practices her new skills in bed," explains Dr. T. Berry Brazelton. Expect further disturbances around age 9 months. "A baby who is learning to get up to standing will practice at night, too. When put to bed, she'll stand up in the crib as soon as the parent leaves the room. If you put her down, up she comes again—10 times or more."

Around the time of your child's first birthday, you can again anticipate some backsliding. "There is a rapid increase in cognitive awareness (of strangers or strange situations, of new places, of changes in the daily routine) that coincide with spurts in motor development (walking, climbing). The excitement and fears this generates may temporarily interrupt a child's sleep patterns," Dr. Brazelton says.

- *Stress.* When life becomes too challenging, it's tempting for a toddler or preschooler to back away and become a baby again—and to him, being a baby may mean fussing at bedtime or crying for comfort in the middle of the night. What constitutes stress, kiddie style? Weaning from the breast or bottle, toilet training, moving to another home, starting daycare or preschool, the birth of a new sibling, a mother's return to work, or any major family upset such as a divorce or death of a loved one can all be stressful.

Thalia Davis can attest to that: "My husband and I separated 4 months ago, and our 2½-year-old son has become quite clingy. Bobby refuses to sleep in his big-boy bed, though when he first got it a year ago, he was excited about it. Instead, he insists on sleeping with me. He even keeps his hand in my hair all night, as if to make sure I can't leave."

• *Illness.* Backsliding is also common whenever a child is sick. "For one thing, she may be too uncomfortable to sleep soundly. She's likely to wake during the night and need some extra soothing in order to get back to sleep," explains Dr. Deborah E. Sewitch. "She soon becomes accustomed to receiving this special attention and is loath to give it up, even after she's well again."

A variety of common illnesses and aches can hinder sleep:

• Colds make it difficult to breathe through the nose, interfering with deep sleep and increasing nighttime wakings.
• Middle-ear pressure can intensify while lying down, so the pain of an ear infection may worsen when the child tries to sleep.

- Teething pain can contribute to bedtime fussiness and nighttime wakings. Discomfort usually lasts 1 or 2 days per tooth, and is more troublesome when several teeth come in simultaneously or in rapid succession.
- Croup, an infection of the voice box that is accompanied by a distinctive barking-seal cough, often comes on suddenly in the night and lasts up to 6 days.
- Stomachaches can interfere with sleep, especially among children who have food sensitivities of which parents are unaware. A child who is allergic to eggs, for instance, may be kept awake by a tummyache after eating an omelet for dinner.
- Sore throat due to strep or another infection may make a child too uncomfortable to sleep well until the problem is diagnosed and appropriate treatment begun.

When your child is ill or in pain, discuss the situation with your pediatrician. She can recommend over-the-counter or prescription medications, dietary changes, and other techniques for alleviating the symptoms. Soon your little one should be feeling—and sleeping—better.

How to Keep a Temporary Regression from Becoming an Entrenched Habit

"When a child experiences an illness, difficult developmental stage, or traumatic life event, he often will seek comfort in the night. This is a sign of normal emotional regression, and you can certainly give him the comfort he needs," notes Dr. Charles E. Schaefer. "But be careful to keep this from turning back into a habit. Many children see once as an exception but twice as the new rule."

Just how do you nip a re-emerging pattern in the bud? Tackle the backsliding with the same strategy you used to correct the problem initially. Within 1 to 3 nights, your child should remember her old sleep training and settle back into more acceptable behavior. "Leah got a bad stomach flu when she was 13 months old, and for a week she could tolerate nothing but breastmilk. I'd put her to bed at her usual time, but she'd wake up starving every night and want a full feeding. Because I was concerned that she was so uncomfortable and was getting little to eat, I went ahead and nursed her," says Amy Marz, mother of two girls. "After 10 nights of this, her virus was gone—but her midnight snacking habit was back in full force, just as it had been before I'd broken her of it 6 months earlier. I said to myself, 'Uh-oh, I've seen this movie before and I didn't like it then. No way am I going to sit through a double feature.' I used the cold-turkey approach again, and within a couple of nights, Leah was sleeping through with no more complaints."

ROOMMATES, WOMBMATES, BABYSITTERS, JET-SETTERS, AND OTHER SITUATIONS THAT CAN COMPLICATE SLEEP ROUTINES

Sleep-training techniques that seem sensible for handling a single child in your own home can become unwieldy when conditions are less than ideal. Here's how to succeed under complicated circumstances.

When Siblings Share Sleeping Quarters

"On nights when 4-year-old Kelsey doesn't want to go to sleep at bedtime, she knows just what to do. She makes such a fuss that I'm afraid she'll wake her baby sister, with whom she shares a room," says Jennifer Trillo, mother of three girls, with a sigh. "Kelsey has figured out that I'll do almost anything, including let her stay up late, to keep her quiet so the baby can sleep. It's a real problem, because I feel there's no way I can enforce bedtime."

Jennifer is all too familiar with a fact of life many parents of two or more kids can verify: sleep-training techniques are far trickier to implement when two siblings are sharing a bedroom. How can you let a 12-month-old cry it out without disturbing his big brother? Is it fair to use the door-closing method to control a preschooler's nighttime wanderings, since you'd also be closing the door on her cooperative little sister?

The best bet is to allow the well-behaved sibling to sleep in a separate room until the other child's nighttime behavior has improved. (This way, Kelsey Trillo's bedtime protests would lose their power to strike fear in her mother's heart.) Don't move the disruptive child out instead; it's far more effective for her to undergo her sleep training in the same environment in which she will be expected to sleep in the future. However, do take care not to make this arrangement so pleasant for the cooperative child that she insists on staying in her temporary quarters long after the original problem is solved.

AGE FLAG: NEWBORN TO 4 MONTHS

One possible exception to this rule is when the disruptive child is an infant. Because she needs to be fed around the clock, you can't "train" her not to create a disturbance at night. At this tender age, she is probably not as acutely aware of her environment as an older child would be. "If the infant's cries wake up her roommate, temporarily move the baby's bassinet into the hall or put her to sleep in her playpen in the living room. Once she's sleeping more soundly at night, you can move her back into the shared bedroom," suggests Dr. Deborah Madansky.

Sometimes just a bit of reassurance can quickly ease a roommate back to sleep. "Six-year-old Lily has night terrors during which she shouts and rolls around. This wakes up 8-year-old Kimberly, with whom she shares a room," says Rose Mary Wood, mother of 14 children. "Whenever it happens, I go into the girls' bedroom and reassure Kimberly that her sister is all right. At that point, Kim usually goes right back to sleep in her own bed, even if Lily's still yelling."

Another common conflict between roommates occurs when one sibling regularly gets out of his own bed in the middle of the night and climbs into bed next to his brother, disturbing the second sibling's sleep. Try moving the children's beds closer together so the wandering child feels more secure about his brother's presence. Or place a sleeping bag on the floor next to the second child's bed; tell the wandering child that he may sleep there if he wishes, but that he must not wake up his sibling by getting into bed with him.

Or perhaps your problem occurs in the morning, when one child habitually wakes up earlier than the other and then proceeds to bother her still-slumbering sibling. If your early bird's a baby, you may need to anticipate her 5 A.M. cry and set your alarm so you can fetch her and feed her at the first peep. With an older early riser, teach the child to look at books in bed or to play quietly in the family room until the rest of the clan is up. Make it clear that she may not talk or play loudly in the bedroom until her roommate is awake.

Same or Separate Bedtimes for Siblings?

Deciding whether to put your children to bed at the same time or at different times may require a bit of experimentation, as well as an evaluation of each child's sleep needs.

When children are more than a couple years apart in age, it makes sense to put the youngest to bed first. Enjoy an age-appropriate bedtime routine with him, then once he's settled down, spend some one-on-one time with your older child as she prepares for bed. In this arrangement, you may find advantages that go beyond a conflict-free bedtime, as my sister Barbara Eberlein did. "I think having a later bedtime helps my son keep his feelings of sibling rivalry in check. He appreciates the fact that his little sister, who's nearly 3 years younger, will be put to bed first, and that then he and I will have some private time together."

On the other hand, when kids are close in age, it

may be more convenient to get them all ready for bed at the same time, and let everybody participate in a big family-style bedtime routine. Then tuck each child in individually, spending a few private minutes talking and cuddling with each one. This schedule suits me well. Since my youngest boy is just 2 years younger than my twins, all the kids have lights-out at the same time. To make up for the additional rest he needs, little Jack typically sleeps an hour later in the morning.

Twins and Sleep: Avoiding Double Trouble

Some parents of twins are happy to have their babies on different sleep schedules. "Taking care of just one baby while the other sleeps is less chaotic, plus it allows you one-on-one time with each child," notes British pediatrician Elizabeth M. Bryan, M.D., author of *Twins, Triplets and More.*

That's how I felt—in the beginning. But after a month or so, I realized that with my twins on different daytime and nighttime schedules, one baby was always awake and in need of me. I had not a moment to myself. At that point, establishing a coordinated schedule became a priority.

If you feel as I did, you can begin by keeping a sleep diary for each baby, then examine the logs for any similarities. My records helped me see that both my babies typically napped for 2 hours in the morning, but James fell asleep at 10:30 and Samantha at 11:30. I postponed his nap by actively entertaining him for half an hour, and moved hers up to 11:00 by cutting short the midmorning play and rocking her instead. It didn't always work, of course—you can't expect babies to be like Swiss watches—but on those occasions when I did manage to get both down for a nap at once, I had time for a quick shower or much-needed snooze.

In the evening, get your twins ready for bed at the same time. "To help get our infant twins on the same schedule, we established a nightly routine of bath-bottle-bed. The girls were down by 8 P.M. every evening, giving my husband and me some adult time," notes Kelly Kassab, who is the mother of three.

Some sociable twins who are put to bed together keep each other awake with chattering or crying. If this is a habitual problem in your family, consider staggering the twins' bedtimes slightly. Lisa McDonough, a mother of four, explains, "Whenever I tried to put my 1-year-olds to bed at the same time, they yelled across the room to each other for what seemed like an hour. Now I put Meghan down 20 minutes earlier, so she's asleep before Kevin goes into his crib."

Can twins share a crib? That can work for the first 3 months, but then it gets overcrowded. As for sharing a bedroom, it depends. "Some twins sleep through each other's cries, while others wake at their partner's first whimper," says Dr. Bryan. This mutual awakening isn't necessarily bad if you're working toward a shared schedule. But when room sharing causes constant disturbances, put the twins in different bedrooms or let them take turns sleeping in the living room.

AGE FLAG: NEWBORN TO 4 MONTHS

As for double disturbances in the middle of the night, they're inevitable at first because the babies will need to eat. As a general rule, I'm in favor of feeding on demand, but with twins, you have to compromise a bit on those nighttime feedings. If you allow the babies total control over the schedule, you may find yourself feeding the first one at 1 A.M. and the second at 2:30—which means that, by 4 A.M., the first one will be hungry again, and so you'll never get more than an hour of uninterrupted sleep. To prevent this problem, do your best to wake the second twin to feed with or immediately after the first. If you can master the fine art of simultaneously feeding twins at the breast or bottle, feedings will go far more quickly and you'll get back to bed that much faster.

Once the twins reach 3 months, however, one if not both may be ready to sleep 5 or 6 hours at a stretch. At that point, experiment for a few nights to see what happens if you don't wake that second twin along with the first. If she screams to be fed half an hour after you've put her sister back to bed, go back to feeding them together for a few more weeks. But if you're lucky, baby number two will sleep through the night— and you'll be halfway home to a full night's sleep yourself.

When the Babysitter's in Charge of Bedtime

The first rule for ensuring that the evening goes smoothly in your absence is to let the child meet and get comfortable with any new babysitter before you leave the house. If your date is a late one, you may be tempted to prevent any protests by putting the child to bed yourself, then departing after he's asleep. But this is a near-guarantee of trouble, warns Dr. Sewitch. "An infant may not be upset if an unfamiliar caregiver answers his awakening cry, but any child over age 6 months is likely to feel extremely fearful if she cries out during the night for her mother and instead is confronted with a sitter whom she's never met."

If the babysitter will be handling the sleep preparations on her own, you need to review with her every aspect of your child's regular bedtime ritual. Explain the order in which tasks such as teeth brushing and putting on pajamas are performed. Tell her how many stories you usually read and which songs you always sing. Let her know whether your child customarily sleeps with a night light on, with the draperies drawn, and with the bedroom door open or closed. Be certain she understands that your child is encouraged to sleep with his lovey, and verify that this object is in the child's bed or in his arms before you leave the house—because nothing hurls bedtime into chaos quite the way a lost lovey does.

"If possible, have a new sitter drop by your house for an hour at bedtime a day or two before you plan to go out. She can help you put the child to bed and get some hands-on experience with your unique routine," suggests Dr. Sewitch. This not only allows the sitter and the child to feel more comfortable doing the ritual in your absence, but also lessens the likelihood that the kid will get away with hours of stalling by pretending that "Mom always reads me 15 books before bed."

It's not necessary for absolutely every aspect of your child's bedtime routine to be reproducible by a babysitter, so long as most aspects are. For instance, my kids know that the sitter can provide the customary camel ride into the bathroom, assist with teeth brushing and putting on P.J.s, read two books of the children's choice, and sing the "I Love You" song. But they also know that she will not sing the "Te Amo" song in Spanish, or add another episode to our ongoing epic of "James, Samantha, and Jack and the Magic Flying Blankies." They accept these omissions with good grace on the evenings I'm not at home, provided I tell the blankie story earlier in the day.

If your babysitter is a live-in nanny who often puts your child to bed, it's vital that she share your views (or at least comply with your instructions) on how to deal with bedtime protests and middle-of-the-night disturbances. Otherwise, your child may become confused by the mixed messages she receives, and the effectiveness of any sleep-training methods you implement may be compromised.

Is your child prone to nightmares, night terrors, or sleepwalking? (More on sleepwalking later in this chapter.) If so, familiarize each of your babysitters—and the parents of playmates who invite your youngster to sleep over—with these phenomena, and explain how episodes can best be handled. Forgetting to do this could place your child at risk for emotional upset or even physical injury.

Daycare providers, too, may need to be kept apprised of your child's sleep problems. For example, if your youngster simply isn't tired at bedtime, it could be that he's napping too long at daycare. Find out how much rest time is scheduled during the day; if it seems excessive, ask the staff to cut the total naptime down and to eliminate any late-afternoon naps completely. Working together, you and the caregivers can do much to assure a good night's sleep for your child.

Sleep Tips for Traveling Tots

It's an unfortunate fact that sleep disruptions are virtually unavoidable when kids are put to bed in an unfamiliar hotel room or on Grandma's lumpy sofa bed, but there are steps you can take to minimize the problems.

Begin even before you leave home. If during the trip your baby will be sleeping in a portable crib, set the crib up at home a few days in advance, and let him "practice" napping there. When you pack, include your baby's customary crib blanket. Help an older child pack her own special "bedtime bag" with everything she'll need for her nightly routine: toothbrush, toothpaste, comb, brush, pajamas, favorite books, night light, small toys to play with in bed, even a tape player and tapes if these are part of the usual bedtime ritual. But don't put her lovey away in a suitcase; instead, keep it handy for encouraging naps in her carseat or on board the airplane.

Once you've arrived, try to maintain the child's normal schedule as much as possible. He's more likely to sleep well if he's not kept up long past his usual bedtime. But of course, sometimes delays are unavoidable. "Don't be so rigid about bedtime that it interferes with the fun of the trip. The schedule police aren't going to give you a ticket if you let your child stay up an hour or two later while on vacation," says Dr. Martin Scharf.

If you have crossed time zones, your child's schedule (and your own) may be out of whack. Help her adjust to the new time over the next several nights. The procedure for doing so depends on which direction you've flown:

- *East to west.* Suppose your child normally hits the hay at 8 P.M. Eastern time. Now that she's arrived on the West Coast, she may feel sleepy by 5 P.M., and thus miss out on the evening activity. Even worse, her Eastern-time internal clock may awaken her as usual at 7 A.M.—even though the Pacific-time clock on the nightstand says 4 A.M.

  To prevent these problems, try to keep your child up until 6 o'clock that first evening, suggests Dr. Sewitch. When she wakes the next morning, probably around 5 A.M., encourage her to read or play quietly in bed for an hour. Delay breakfast as long as possible so her other body rhythms start to move into sync with the local schedule. Put her to bed at 7 o'clock that second night, anticipating a 6 A.M. awakening. By the third night, she should be ready for an 8 o'clock lights-out and a 7 A.M. Pacific-time reveille.

- *West to east.* The California kid whose normal bedtime is 8 o'clock is unlikely to be tired at 8 P.M. on her first night in New York, since her internal clock is telling her it's only 5 P.M. "Let her stay up until 10 o'clock the first night, and until 9 the second night. By the third night, she should be ready for bed by 8 o'clock," Dr. Sewitch says. If she has any trouble falling asleep during this adjustment period, let her look at books or play quietly in bed until she feels tired.

Once you've returned home, get right back into your regular routine. If jet lag's a problem, you can ease your child into the normal home schedule over several nights, as described above. But beyond that, don't make any extra allowances in the name of easing her "adjustment." Maybe she did get used to sleeping with Mom and Dad during your stay at Aunt Jennifer's, but now that you're home, she's got her own room once more. If that's where she had been sleeping before your trip, that's where she should sleep again—starting the very first night you're home. "Let her learn to doze off on her own again, in her own room, even if it means putting up with a few more nights of tears," counsels Dr. Madansky. Otherwise, the temporary sleep arrangements that made sense during your trip may become permanent but senseless habits at home.

When Parents Divorce: Sleep Problems to Expect, Routines to Enforce

"My son Bobby was never a good sleeper, but the situation worsened markedly after my husband and I separated," admits Thalia Davis. "Now when Bobby visits his dad for the weekend, he has a very different sleep routine from the one he has with me. I suspect this isn't helping the problem."

Thalia's right. Splitting time between two households can cause or exacerbate a variety of sleep disturbances in children. "To minimize the problems, the most important thing divorced parents can do is come to an agreement on how bedtime and other sleep issues should be handled," urges Dr. Jodi Mindell. This is in your child's best interest—and even if you're agreeing on little else, you'll probably agree on the importance of doing what's best for your child. Try to come to a consensus with your ex on the following matters:

- *Bedtime.* A consistent bedtime in both households helps to minimize the physiological and psychological demands imposed by frequently shuttling back and forth between two abodes.

- *Bedtime ritual.* The rituals practiced by Mom and Dad won't be absolutely identical, of course, but having a number of similarities between the two routines can help the child feel at home in both his bedrooms and provide a sense of familiarity that makes it easier to fall asleep.

- *Lovey.* When a child is adjusting to her parents' split, the last thing she needs is to be denied her adored teddy or favorite blanket. Don't say to her, "That old bunny your father gave you can stay at his apartment; here at home you can sleep with this nice new lamb I bought." Remember, a child's lovey must be an object of her own choosing. Encourage her to carry that bunny back and forth between her two homes, a much-needed constant in her ever-changing world.

- *Sleeping quarters.* If you were advocates of the family bed before the divorce, you can each probably continue to share a bed with your child. But if you're tempted to start cosleeping to dispel your own loneliness, you may be asking for trouble. (Review Chapter Five for guidelines on making this important decision.)

Ideally, both parents should resist the temptation to be the "nice guy" who allows the child to stay up late, get up for a midnight snack, or sneak into the parent's bed at night. Usually it's the noncustodial parent who's more likely to do this, since most of the negative repercussions will be felt by the other parent as she struggles to get the child back into his normal routine. Not only is this unfair to the custodial parent, it's unfair to the child as well—because when his sleep patterns go haywire, he feels the worse for it. (To understand why, review Chapter One.)

AGE FLAG: 2½ YEARS AND UP

If you're the custodial parent and your ex is letting the child get away with bedtime mayhem, you need to be especially committed to maintaining consistent sleep routines when the child's at home. "It's better for the child to have rules and consistency in only one household than to have them in neither," Dr. Sewitch explains. Here's a sample script for getting that message across to your child.

CHILD: Aw, Mom, I don't want to go to bed yet. It's only 8 o'clock.

PARENT: Eight-thirty is your usual bedtime. Let's go into the bathroom together and brush your teeth, and then I'll read to you until it's time for bed.

CHILD: But I'm not tired. I stayed up till 10 o'clock last night, and till 11 the night before, at Dad's house. Dad always lets me stay up late—sometimes till midnight.

PARENT: I know he does, and I don't agree with that, but Dad makes the decisions in his own house. Here, though, I make the rules, and in this house you go to bed at 8:30 so you'll feel rested for school in the morning.

CHILD: You're a meanie. Dad's nicer than you.

PARENT: I'm sorry you feel that way. I'm not trying to be mean. I think one reason Dad lets you stay up late is that on weekends, you don't have to worry about getting up for school. I know it's not easy having to adjust to two different sets of rules. But it's important for you to know what the rules are here at home, and to follow them.

CHILD: But I know I won't be able to fall asleep yet. After spending a weekend at Dad's, I'm just not used to going to bed so early. Let me stay up until 9 o'clock, at least.

PARENT: If you're not tired, you may certainly look at books in bed until you feel sleepy, even if that means you're awake until 9 or even later.

CHILD: Oh, okay. I'll race you into the bathroom!

This parent does a good job of reminding her child of the house rule about bedtime, and explaining why the rule is important. She sticks to her guns even when challenged, without losing her temper or letting the conversation degenerate into hurtful name-calling. She sympathizes with the trouble the youngster is having in adjusting, but doesn't allow that to interfere with the re-establishment of the regular routine. When the child complains that he won't be able to sleep, she offers to let him read in bed until he's tired—a very reasonable compromise.

INFANTS ONLY: THE UNIQUE SLEEP PATTERNS OF PREEMIES

"Push!" my doctor commanded, but I didn't want to push. I didn't want my twins to be born, not yet. "It's too soon; they're too little—they'll die," I cried, but there was no stopping the labor. Nine weeks premature, my 3-pound son and 2-pound daughter entered the world.

My babies spent 5 weeks in intensive care, struggling to survive and learning to do things most newborns do instinctively—things like suck and breathe and keep their hearts beating. No wonder they also had trouble learning to sleep on any sort of a "normal" schedule.

If you've got a preterm infant, accept one important fact: you cannot compare her developmentally to a full-term baby born at the same time. "Until your child is 2 years old, in gauging her development, you must correct for the number of weeks premature she was. For instance, a girl born at 30 weeks' instead of 40 weeks' gestation cannot be fairly compared at 3 months of age with a 3-month-old full-term baby. Subtract the number of weeks early your child was from her chronological age to arrive at her 'corrected age.' Three months after she was born, your baby developmentally is about 2 weeks old," explains Jessie R. Groothuis, M.D., professor of pediatrics at the University of Colorado School of Medicine. In other words, don't expect your preemie to sleep through the night at 3 or 4 months of age; developmentally, she's unlikely to be ready for that until she's about 6 months old.

Another way in which prematurity affects sleep has to do with a preemie's nutritional needs. Premature babies need to eat more often. When my twins were discharged from the hospital, they weighed just over 4 pounds. No way could their tiny tummies hold enough milk to carry them through for 4 hours, so I was given strict instructions to feed them every 2 hours. Not until their weight had climbed to about 9 pounds did my pediatrician give me the go-ahead to stretch feedings to every 3 to 4 hours. Until that happened, catnaps were the order of my children's day (and night).

Preemies are also more likely to mix up their days and nights. This is due in part to the fact that, in the hospital, certain routine procedures such as bathing are often performed on the late-night shift. By the time your preemie comes home, he may be used to snoozing the day away and splashing around at midnight. (To reverse this pattern, refer to Chapter Three's Infants Only section for tips on helping baby differentiate daytime and nighttime.)

You also may have to put some extra effort into helping your preemie adjust to a dark, quiet nursery. The first evening my infant daughter was home from the hospital, after all the well-wishers had departed, I sat with her in the nursery and quietly rocked her as I watched the sunlight fade. It dawned on me then that little Samantha had never before seen darkness or heard silence. The neonatal intensive care unit had been a brightly lit ward filled with beeping vital-signs monitors, constant conversation, and the echoes of the tiny patients' cries.

If your preemie seems fretful in the unfamiliar quietude of home, try leaving a light on in her room. Near her crib, place a radio, ticking clock, or tape player with a recording of hospital sounds. Then over the next week or so, gradually dim the light and turn down the sound, until your baby adapts to a more tranquil way of life.

SLEEP DISORDERS: SELF-HELP AND PROFESSIONAL HELP

Sleep disorders are physical or psychological problems that cause a person to lose sleep and suffer excessive daytime sleepiness. The most common ones affecting children are sleepwalking, sleep apnea, insomnia, and bedwetting. Sometimes the situation can be handled at home as you wait for the child to outgrow the behavior; in serious or persistent cases, a doctor should be consulted.

When a Child Sleepwalks

AGE FLAG: 3 TO 8 YEARS

Technically called somnambulism, sleepwalking is common among preschool and early school-age children, with up to 40 percent of youngsters experiencing at least one episode. Boys are more often affected than girls. The tendency is hereditary; if either parent was a sleepwalker, a child is 6 to 10 times more likely to sleepwalk as well.

Often, it's tricky to recognize sleepwalking for what it is; parents may think their child is simply being difficult or disobedient. In fact, one sleep expert interviewed for this book confessed with embarrassment that the first time his own daughter went wandering, he did not realize she was sleepwalking until his wife suggested that as a possible explanation for the child's queer behavior.

Most sleepwalking episodes occur within 1 to 3 hours after a child falls asleep, and last from 5 to 20 minutes. In its most mild form, sleepwalking consists of sitting up in bed and mumbling. More complex forms involve leaving the bed and roaming around inside or even outside the house. The child moves clumsily, yet often manages to negotiate stairways and find his way around furniture. He may perform simple tasks like opening and closing drawers or doors, getting and eating food, going to the bathroom, and turning on lights. He may engage in bizarre behavior, such as urinating in a closet or wastebasket. His eyes are probably open but appear unfocused; his face most likely is expressionless. If he responds to other people at all, it is with simple one- or two-word replies.

Kelly Dunkin, a mother of two, has been living with a sleepwalker for several years. "My daughter Kaeri started sleepwalking at age 3. She had an episode almost every night—sometimes two or three per night—for about 6 months, then it started tapering off. Now she's 5, and she still sleepwalks once or twice a week," explains Kelly. "Often she walks downstairs as if she's looking for someone, with her eyes half open. Sometimes she's crying, and other times she's silent."

Somnambulism is believed to be the result of an immature central nervous system. Like night terrors, it is a disorder of arousal; physiologically, there is a simultaneous occurrence of partial wakefulness and non-REM sleep as a child starts to make the transition from deep sleep to the lighter-sleep dream state of REM.

This is not to say that there's truth to the old myth about a sleepwalker "acting out his dreams," however. For one thing, the child is not yet dreaming when the sleepwalking begins. What's more, during REM sleep (when dreaming occurs) a person's muscles are virtually paralyzed, except for those controlling the diaphragm and eye movements. It would be quite impossible for a person who's dreaming to wander around the house.

A sleepwalking episode can be triggered by a variety of factors. Fatigue is a primary contributor. Dr. Schaefer explains, "The biochemical response to sleep loss includes the release of adrenaline and noradrenaline, stimulating chemicals that fight fatigue and upset sleep patterns. This can extend the amount of time spent in sleep stages three and four, and thus increase the likelihood of sleepwalking." A noctural walk also may be sparked by a high fever. Although fever initially suppresses deep sleep, this suppression is later followed by a rebound-type increase in stage-three and -four sleep that makes the child more prone to a partial arousal. In fact, anything that increases his time spent in deep sleep—apprehension, illness, pain, certain medications—also increases the likelihood of a sleepwalking episode.

This does not mean that only stressful or unpleasant experiences trigger sleepwalking; excitement often does, too. "Kaeri inevitably has an episode when we're staying overnight at Grandma's house, and on the first night after we come home," Kelly reports.

The first question many parents ask when they learn

their child sleepwalks is, "Is it true that you should never wake a sleepwalker?" That's good advice, some experts say. "It's dangerous to try to wake a sleepwalking adult because his behavior may become extraordinarily, even primitively violent," Dr. Scharf explains. "With a child, there's less of a threat because you can overwhelm him physically, but still there's no point in risking having him get out of control."

Other sleep researchers theorize that waking a sleepwalker is actually beneficial because it allows him to start a sleep cycle afresh. And still others claim there's neither risk nor benefit to attempting to wake him, but that you're unlikely to succeed in doing so.

If you feel you must rouse a sleepwalker because she's in danger, simply repeat her name calmly until she shows signs of responding. Do not yell, slap or shake her, or splash cold water on her face. If the child is very agitated, do not attempt to restrain her unless she appears to be headed for danger; this could upset her further. "Sometimes when I try to take Kaeri back to bed, she screams and breaks away from me, and then runs into a corner as if she's trying to hide," says Kelly. If this happens, wait a few minutes. Once the child calms down, you should be able to gently lead her back to bed.

The following morning, your child will probably have no memory of the event, although he may remember waking up later in a room other than the one in which he went to sleep. Do not alarm him with an interrogation or expressions of deep concern. "If you consider sleepwalking to be abnormal and frightening, so will your child; if you consider it a normal part of maturation, so will he," says Dr. Schaefer.

For parents of a sleepwalker, the first priority must be the child's safety. You need to get up and be with her whenever an episode occurs. Use a nursery monitor to wake you when she gets up, or attach a bell or battery-operated alarm to her doorknob so you'll know when she leaves her room. Before you go to sleep each night, your house must be sleepwalker-proofed.

"To keep Kaeri from tripping, my husband and I make sure the hallways are well lit and free of clutter, and that there are no electrical cords sticking out. We put all sharp objects out of reach. We place a gate across the top of the stairway and lock the windows. And we've installed special locks on all the outside doors, to make certain Kaeri can't open them and wander out," explains Kelly.

You can minimize the number of sleepwalking episodes your child has by guarding against fatigue. Make sure he goes to bed at a reasonable hour, especially when ill or overtired. If naps were recently abandoned without good reason, reinstitute them. Another effective approach is the prompted-awakenings method also used to prevent night terrors. (See the Chapter Four section called "Prevention Tactics for Night Terrors" for a detailed description.) In brief, you keep a sleep log for a week or so, recording how many minutes elapse from the time your child falls asleep until the time the sleepwalking episode begins. Once you've found the pattern, awaken your child 15 minutes before the anticipated start of the sleepwalking, and keep him fully awake for 5 minutes. Do this for 7 consecutive nights, then stop. If the sleepwalking continues, repeat the 7-night program of prompted awakenings.

For many children, this approach significantly reduces the number of episodes they experience.

Most children outgrow sleepwalking before they reach adolescence, and medical treatment usually is not required. However, if the episodes occur several times a night, if the child exhibits extremely agitated or violent behavior, or if the sleepwalking is causing severe disruption in the family, it's time to get professional help. Treatment options include psychotherapy, hypnosis, and medication that decreases the time spent in the deepest stages of sleep.

The Risks of Sleep Apnea

Sleep apnea is a pause in breathing of more than 10 seconds that occurs repeatedly when a person is asleep. "Apnea disrupts sleep because each time it occurs, the body is deprived of oxygen and the sleeper partially awakes in an effort to resume breathing. In severe cases, sleep clinicians have recorded as many as 319 episodes of apnea during 7 hours of sleep," reports Dr. Schaefer. Although the person begins to breathe again shortly after each apnic pause, his sleep is interrupted so frequently that he is unable to get enough deep sleep, so he never feels well rested.

A child with sleep apnea may exhibit the following symptoms:

• Frequent pauses in breathing during sleep that last more than 10 seconds
• Recurrent episodes of waking and gasping for breath
• Chronic loud snoring or labored breathing at night

- Mouth breathing
- Extreme restlessness during sleep
- Recurrent infections of the upper respiratory tract
- Morning headaches
- Chronic daytime drowsiness
- Chronic irritability, lack of self-control, poor concentration, or other signs of sleep deprivation (see Chapter One for a complete list).

Sleep apnea is most common among children who have enlarged tonsils and/or adenoids that block air passages. Being overweight can compound the problem, but will not in itself cause sleep apnea.

If you suspect your child may have sleep apnea, consult your pediatrician; she can refer you to an appropriate specialist. A commonly recommended treatment is surgical removal of the enlarged tonsils and adenoids, to open the upper airway. "This is one of the few reasons surgeons perform tonsillectomies anymore, and it's an important one," says Dr. Sewitch.

If the doctor determines that a child's overbite is contributing to the problem, a plastic dental appliance called a modified mandibular repositioner can open the airway by moving the lower jaw forward. In some cases, a doctor may recommend a continuous positive airway pressure device, or CPAP device. This triangular mask fits over the nose and helps to regulate air flow. Fortunately, sleep apnea usually disappears when the underlying condition is detected and treated.

Insomnia: When Kids Can't Sleep

Suppose your child tosses and turns in bed for half an hour or more each night. It's not that she's rebelling against bedtime; she simply can't seem to doze off. Or perhaps she often wakes up long before dawn. She doesn't call out for comforting or attention; she simply stares at the ceiling for an hour before finally falling back to sleep. If either of these scenarios sounds familiar, your child may have insomnia.

There are a number of reasons why a child may have trouble falling or staying asleep night after night, and likewise a number of ways in which parents can help solve the problem. Here are some suggestions:

- Be sure her bedtime is appropriate. "You can't send a 5-year-old to bed at 6:30 and expect her to go right to sleep," notes Dr. May Griebel. Review the Chapter One section called "How Much Is a Kid Supposed to Sleep, Anyway?" to determine whether your estimate of your child's sleep needs is realistic or excessive. Also consider the possibility that your youngster is a "short sleeper"—one who needs less sleep than average. Dr. Griebel says, "If she tosses and turns for an hour before dropping off, yet appears alert and well rested during the day, you're probably putting her to bed too early." The easy fix: move her bedtime back.

- Don't let him sleep late in the morning, even if you're worried that he didn't get enough rest during the night. Why not? Because sleeping late sets the stage for another bout of insomnia the following night. If the child takes forever to fall asleep and then is extremely difficult to awaken in the morning, he may have a sleep phase delay rather than true insomnia. For help, refer to the Chapter One section called "How to Handle a Night Owl."

· Avoid overstimulation in the hour before bedtime. A child who's wound up after an extra-exciting evening may have to lie in bed a long time waiting for his body and brain to settle down. Replace after-dinner tickle games and pillow fights with calmer activities like board games, books, and puzzles. On those nights when excitement is inevitable—after a suppertime birthday celebration, for example—extend the bedtime ritual slightly to give the child extra time to calm down before being tucked in.

· How about that age-old remedy for insomnia, a glass of warm milk? It's worth a try. Milk contains the amino acid tryptophan, which is converted by the brain into serotonin. Because this chemical has a calming effect, it makes some people feel drowsy. But in other people, the opposite effect may occur because milk is also high in protein, which sparks production of the energizing brain chemicals dopamine and norepinephrine. "If milk before bed revs up your youngster, try giving him a light snack of bread, cereal, rice cakes, or crackers. Carbohydrate foods such as these also trigger production of soothing serotonin, as milk does, but without the added protein punch," suggests Michael Stevenson, Ph.D., clinical director of the North Valley Sleep Disorders Center in Mission Hills, California.

· What you don't want to include in that bedtime snack, or even the after-school snack, is any caffeine. "Caffeine is a very long-acting drug. Even a midafternoon cola can interfere with sleep that night," explains Dr. Griebel. If your child seems at all sensitive to caffeine, restrict consumption of cola, tea, and cocoa to lunchtime or earlier.

- Insomnia can be a sign that the child is struggling with some troubling emotional issue. If your child seems generally anxious, try to get her to talk to you about whatever might be bothering her—problems with a playmate, stress at school, rivalry with a sibling, worries about the family—so you can work out a solution together.

- Some parents try to treat insomnia by giving the child an over-the-counter antihistamine to make him drowsy. But this is a one-night quick-fix at best, not a permanent solution to the underlying problem. If you can't figure out what's keeping your youngster awake night after night, don't just drug him; take him to a doctor.

"All children (and adults) have trouble sleeping sometimes, so you needn't fret over an occasional wakeful night," says Dr. Sewitch. "But if the problem persists, occurring nearly every night for several weeks or showing any type of repetitive pattern, it's time to seek professional help." Consult your pediatrician first; if necessary, he can refer you to a specialist.

Battling Bedwetting

Sleep specialists view bedwetting as a disorder only when it continues past age 5. For children not yet old enough for kindergarten, few experts would recommend any treatment beyond the self-help measures outlined below. By first grade, however, a child who has not yet outgrown bedwetting may indeed benefit from professional help.

Bedwetting affects approximately 1 in 3 4-year-olds, with boys outnumbering girls. It is common even among preschoolers who achieved good daytime bladder control months or years earlier. By 6 years of age, 10 percent of children have not yet outgrown the problem. Among 10-year-olds, consistent nighttime dryness is still an elusive goal for 1 in 20 youngsters.

Heredity is perhaps the single most important factor in determining who wets the bed. If one of his parents was a bedwetter in childhood, a youngster has a 45 percent chance of developing the problem; if both parents were bedwetters, there's a 75 percent chance that their child will be, too.

Traditionally, persistent bedwetting has been thought of as an emotional problem. However, it is now known that biological factors play a much greater role than do psychological factors. Many bedwetters have bladders with a smaller-than-average capacity, even if the bladder itself is of normal size. In such children, the sensation of needing to urinate occurs more frequently, even when the bladder is not completely full. In addition, some researchers theorize that bedwetters may sleep more deeply than nonwetters, while others believe that wetters are simply less adept at waking from deep sleep in response to the bladder's signal of fullness. Bedwetters also may produce more urine during the night than the average child, due to insufficient production of the antidiuretic hormone (ADH).

Now that you understand the biological basis behind bedwetting, you will also appreciate the inappropriateness of punishing, scolding, or belittling a child who wets the bed. "A child does not wet the bed out of laziness or naughtiness, and he most certainly would stop if he could," Dr. Stephen Sheldon points out. In fact, a parent who shames or reprimands a child for wetting the bed is likely to find the situation getting worse, as the child's self-esteem plummets and he loses confidence in his ability to tackle the problem.

AGE FLAG: 5 YEARS AND UP

So if your child is under the age of 5, back off a bit and bide your time. Chances are, he'll outgrow the problem. If he doesn't, and the bedwetting persists into kindergarten or beyond, try these strategies:

- Limit liquids in the evening. Let the child drink as much as he wants during the day and through dinnertime, but after that, no more—or at least not more than a few sips.
- Have the child avoid cola, tea, cocoa, and chocolate; all contain caffeine, which is a diuretic.
- Schedule evening bathroom trips, one about 30 minutes before bedtime, and another right before he's tucked in. But don't wake the child up and escort him to the bathroom at your own bedtime, Dr. Sheldon says. "This is treating the bed, not the problem. The bed stays dry, but the child does not learn how to awaken in response to fullness signals from his bladder."

- During the day or as part of the bedtime routine, run through "dry bed exercises." Dr. Sheldon explains: "The child climbs into bed and pretends to be sleeping. After a minute, he pretends to feel the urge to use the toilet, then pretends to wake up, so he gets out of bed and goes to the bathroom." The point of this exercise is to familiarize the child with the routine of leaving his bed, walking down the hall, and using the toilet.
- Praise the child for any dry nights. Praise her, too, whenever she cooperates with the strategies above. You might set up a star chart for recording and rewarding her efforts and especially her successes.
- Let the child share responsibility for the cleanup. You can't insist that a 5-year-old strip her own bed, put on the clean sheets, and launder the soiled ones, but she can help you perform all these chores. Do the job matter-of-factly, with an atmosphere of cooperation and mutual concern—not with recrimination or punishment. To make the task easier, use only machine-washable bedding, and place a waterproof pad beneath the bottom sheet so you won't have to air out the mattress.
- Don't treat the child like a baby by forcing her to wear diapers or plastic pants, or by refusing to allow her to sleep in a regular bed.

What about those ultra-absorbant disposable training pants? The jury is out. "My 4½-year-old son still wets the bed every night. Our pediatrician said the only way Garvey would learn to stay dry was if I put him to bed in regular underpants, so that he'd feel cold and uncomfortable whenever he wet. But still Garv kept wetting the bed, and the workload for me was overwhelming—changing and laundering all those sheets, drying out the mattress," laments Judy Dooley, a mother of four.

Judy decided to use disposable training pants instead. "The problem is, those things are so absorbant that Garv doesn't even realize when they're wet. I ask him in the morning if he's dry, and he says, 'Yes, Mommy,' even though his pants are so soaked with urine that they weigh 20 pounds. What's worse, he feels it's perfectly okay not to use the toilet when he's got his training pants on. One night as I was reading him a bedtime story, I reminded him that if he needed to go potty in the middle of the night, he should get up and go. 'You realize you don't have to pee-pee in your training pants, don't you?' I asked. And then he hung his head and confessed, 'I already did.' While he was wide awake! I was so discouraged. With those pants, Garvey has no motivation to use the toilet when he's awake, much less when he's asleep, but without the pants, life is such a hassle." Judy has chosen a sensible strategy: to continue to use the training pants until her son is 5, hoping he'll outgrow his bedwetting. If he doesn't, she'll take more aggressive action to solve the problem.

That action might eventually include professional help, appropriate for any child 5 to 6 years or older who still wets the bed more than once a week. First, consult your pediatrician; she'll want to rule out any medical causes for the bedwetting, such as a urinary tract infection, diabetes, or urological abnormalities.

The pediatrician or a sleep specialist may then instruct the child to do bladder training exercises (similar to the Kegel exercises taught in childbirth preparation classes). "For instance, when the child goes to the bathroom during the day, he practices stopping his urine flow when his bladder is only half empty. He holds the remaining urine in for a count of five, then finishes voiding," explains Dr. Sheldon. "This helps the child gain more control over his urine stream, and strengthens the muscles that surround the bladder outlet."

Another technique that doctors find effective in many cases is a buzzer system. Consisting of a pad that's placed on the sheet or a sensor worn on the underwear, these systems detect wetness and immediately set off a buzzing alarm as soon as the child begins to urinate. "The system works on the theory that your child will then learn to associate the feelings she has just before urinating with the need to wake up," explains Dr. Richard Ferber.

Children who do not produce adequate amounts of ADH, the purpose of which is to limit urine production during sleep, may benefit from the use of a nasal spray called DDAVP. A synthetic form of ADH, it is available by prescription only.

One highly controversial drug used to control intractable bedwetting is imipramine (Tofranil). "Although when taken in appropriate doses this medicine is relatively safe, it is a powerful drug, and so is no longer commonly used to treat bedwetting. Overdoses can be fatal," warns Dr. Ferber. If your doctor recommends imipramine, discuss the benefits and risks with him in great detail; you need to be fully informed as to the dangers. Dr. Sheldon adds, "I've only used this medicine once in my 20-year career, since the risks are potentially so terribly grave. After all, no child ever died from bedwetting."

Finding Professional Help for Your Child's Sleep Problem

Here are some guidelines on when to get professional help:

* Any time you suspect a physical problem is underlying your child's sleep problem
* When a sleep disturbance interferes with your child's normal daytime behavior for more than 2 weeks
* When a sleep problem is adversely affecting the child's relationship with his parents, peers, caregivers, or teachers
* When the problem is growing worse despite your efforts to correct it
* If you and your spouse cannot agree on how to handle the situation, and this is causing tension in your family

Consult your pediatrician or family physician first about any sleep problem. She will need to review your child's medical history, discuss any symptoms, and perform a complete physical examination. If the doctor suspects that an underlying medical condition is disturbing the child's sleep, she'll conduct tests to confirm the diagnosis and then begin the appropriate treatment. When an emotional problem is indicated, you may be referred to a psychiatrist, psychologist, or social worker. If the doctor concludes that your child has a true sleep disorder or other persistent sleep problem, she may refer you to a sleep disorders center.

WHAT TO EXPECT AT A SLEEP DISORDERS CENTER

When you call to make an appointment at a sleep disorders center, the staff may ask you to keep a detailed log of your child's sleep/wake patterns for 1 or 2 weeks before your first visit. Information they'll request may include the times at which your child goes to bed and wakes up; events that disturb her sleep, and how often and at what time of night they occur; and how your youngster functions during the day. These observations will be of great help as the staff tries to determine the most effective treatment for your child.

During the first appointment, doctors will probably ask you for a complete medical history on your child, then conduct a comprehensive physical and psychological exam. The next step is usually a trial of strategies designed to improve sleep behavior. These will be tailored to suit the individual child and the circumstances of your family.

Some symptoms, such as those suggestive of sleep apnea, may make it advisable for your child to spend 1 or 2 nights in the center's laboratory so his sleep can be monitored. Small sensors placed on the child's head and body record brain waves, muscle activity, leg and arm movements, eye movements, heart rhythms, breathing and other bodily functions as your child sleeps. You will probably be asked to spend the night, too, either in the same room or in another room nearby.

"My kid can't sleep well in his own home. How in the world would he ever fall asleep in a strange laboratory with sensors stuck all over his body?" you might wonder. Fortunately, most kids handle the experience quite well. And the information such a sleep study provides can be invaluable in diagnosing and treating the problem.

———————————— ————————————

Where to Find a Sleep Disorders Center

Need professional help with your youngster's sleep problem? Look for an accredited sleep disorders center that regularly treats children, or better yet, one that specializes in pediatric problems. For a list of centers in your geographical region, write to the National Sleep Foundation, 1367 Connecticut Avenue N.W., Suite 200-TE, Washington, D.C. 20036. Upon request, NSF (which is affiliated with the American Sleep Disorders Association) also provides informational brochures on a variety of sleep problems.

———————————— ✳ ————————————

Final Thoughts

In the weeks after I began researching this book, it seemed as if my own three children were conspiring to force me to learn from personal experience how to handle every sleep problem a parent might encounter. Four-year-old James staged elaborate bedtime rebellions and tried countless tricks to prolong the nightly ritual. His twin sister Samantha, who had always been my best sleeper, suddenly started climbing into bed between me and my husband each night around 3 A.M. Little Jack, 2 years old, experienced his first sleep terror, and then went on to have twice-weekly episodes for months thereafter.

More than once, as we were jarred out of a sound sleep, my husband grumbled to me, "Can't you do something about all this? You're supposed to be the expert. If the situation doesn't improve, even *I'm* not going to buy your book."

Fortunately, the more I learned about children and sleep, the better able I was to handle my own kids' sleep problems. It wasn't always easy, of course. There were some tears, which were heart-wrenching. There was some backsliding, which was discouraging. There were a few out-and-out failures, which were frustrating until I figured out what I was doing wrong and corrected my approach.

But in the end, the results were worth the effort. James started settling down without complaint at bedtime. Samantha learned to stay in her own room, at least until the sun came up. Even Jack's night terrors diminished as I got more proficient at preventing them.

That's not to say that every night is smooth and problem-free now. I don't think any parent can expect perfection when it comes to nighttime behavior, at least not when their children are quite young, but you can expect very significant improvement if you use the methods suggested in this book. You can stop being sleep deprived, and you can stop your children from being sleep deprived, too. You can feel healthier, happier, and more fulfilled as a parent, and your children can feel more content as well. You can get to the point where you go to bed each night fairly confident that you and your kids can sleep undisturbed until morning. And when the sun does come up and your kids bound out of bed, instead of feeling exhausted and intruded upon, you'll be genuinely thrilled to see their smiling faces.

Resources

BOOKS

Brazelton, T. Berry, M.D. *Touchpoints*. Addison-Wesley, 1992

Bryan, Elizabeth M., M.D. *Twins, Triplets and More*. St. Martin's Press, 1992

Cuthbertson, Joanne, and Schevill, Susie. *Helping Your Child Sleep Through the Night*. Doubleday, 1985

Eisenberg, Arlene, Murkoff, Heidi E., and Hathaway, Sandee E., B.S.N. *What to Expect the First Year*. Workman Publishing, 1989

Ferber, Richard, M.D. *Solve Your Child's Sleep Problems*. Fireside, 1985

Huntley, Rebecca. *The Sleep Book for Tired Parents*. City Parenting Press, 1991

Lansky, Vicki. *Getting Your Child to Sleep and Back to Sleep*. The Book Peddlers, 1991

Neidhardt, Joseph, M.D. *Conquering Bad Dreams and Nightmares*. Berkley, 1992

Schaefer, Charles E., Ph.D., and DiGeronimo, Theresa Foy, M.Ed. *Raising Baby Right.* Prince Paperbacks, 1992

Schaefer, Charles E., Ph.D., and DiGeronimo, Theresa Foy, M.Ed. *Winning Bedtime Battles.* Citadel Press, 1992

Scharf, Martin, Ph.D. *Waking Up Dry: How to End Bedwetting Forever.* Writer's Digest, 1986

Schmitt, Barton D., M.D. *Your Child's Health.* Bantam Books, 1991

Sheldon, Stephen, D.O. *Pediatric Sleep Medicine.* W. B. Saunders, 1992

ARTICLES

Barr, Amy Biber. "The Big Switch." *Working Mother,* March, 1994

Chollar, Susan. "Teaching Baby to Sleep Through the Night." *Psychology Today,* April, 1989

Davidowitz, Esther. "Asleep at Last!" *Parents,* July, 1992

Eberlein, Tamara. "Babies Who Go Grunt in the Night." *Redbook,* October, 1991

Eberlein, Tamara. "Does Your Child Wake Up Sweet . . . or Sour?" *Redbook,* October, 1991

Eberlein, Tamara. "Should Your Kids Sleep With You?" *Redbook,* December, 1994

Eberlein, Tamara. "Solve Your Baby's Sleep Problems." *American Baby,* April, 1993

Fahey, Valerie. "I Can't Sleep!" *Sesame Street Parents,* November, 1994

Ferber, Richard, M.D., and Sobel, Dava. "When Your Child Won't Sleep." *Good Housekeeping,* September, 1991

Gibson, Janice T. "A Toddler's Sleep." *Parents,* October, 1988

Graham, Janis. "But I'm Not Sleepy!" *Working Mother,* November, 1994

Graham, Janis. "Negotiating Naptime." *Working Mother,* May, 1994

Greene, Melissa Fay. "A Good Night's Sleep." *Parenting,* May, 1994

Greenspan, Stanley I., M.D. "What Bad Dreams Really Mean." *Parents,* September, 1994

Helligman, Deborah. "How to Handle Nightmares and Night Terrors." *Parents,* November, 1992

Huntley, Rebecca. "Sleep Guide for Tired Parents." *Working Mother,* August, 1992

Jabs, Carolyn. "A Good Night's Sleep." *Working Mother,* February, 1994

Katz, Lillian G., Ph.D. "Nightmares and Other Sleep Problems." *Parents,* April, 1990

Kelly, Jeffrey A. "Bed-wetting." *Parents,* June, 1988

Kelly, Kate Jackson. "The Fear Factor." *Parents,* February, 1994

Klavan, Ellen. "All Through the Night? Not Quite." *Parents,* February, 1987

Lansky, Vicki. "Early Birds." *Sesame Street Parents,* November, 1994

Lansky, Vicki. "Have Blankie, Will Travel." *Sesame Street Parents,* May, 1994

Lawson, Donna. "Will My Child Ever Sleep Through the Night?" *Redbook,* October, 1990

Locker, Hillary. "Sleep Positions." *American Baby,* October, 1994

Marks, Jane. "We Have a Problem: Rachel's Story." *Parents,* September, 1989

Perrone, Janice. "The ABZzzz's of Snoring." *Living Well: The Health News Report,* March, 1993

Rochman, Hazel. "Bedtime Stories." *Sesame Street Parents,* January/February, 1995

Rosemond, John. "Night Terrors." *Better Homes and Gardens,* April, 1993

Schaefer, Charles E., Ph.D., and DiGeronimo, Theresa

Foy. "In Search of Sweet Dreams." *Working Mother,* July, 1994

Schaefer, Charles E., Ph.D., and DiGeronimo, Theresa Foy. "How to Help Your Child Conquer Night Fright." *Redbook,* April, 1992

Segal, Julius, Ph.D., and Segal, Zelda. "Creating a Sleep Routine." *Parents,* March, 1993

Weissbourd, Bernice. "Getting a Good Night's Sleep." *Parents,* March, 1991

Weissbourd, Bernice. "Giving Up Nap Time." *Parents,* November, 1990

Wright, Janice. "Sleep, Little Baby." *American Baby,* May, 1994

Zimmer, Judith. "Children's Sleep Problems: A to ZZZZ." *Redbook,* August, 1993

ORGANIZATIONS

American Academy of Pediatrics
141 Northwest Point Blvd.
Elk Grove Village, IL 60007
(800) 433-9016

American Psychological Association
750 First St. N.E.
Washington, D.C. 20002-4242

National Sleep Foundation
1367 Connecticut Avenue N.W., Suite 200-TE
Washington, D.C. 20036

About the Author

Tamara Eberlein has written over 200 articles on parenting, health, and psychology. Her work has appeared in dozens of national magazines, including *Redbook, Good Housekeeping, Woman's Day, Family Circle, Child, Parents, Parenting, Sesame Street Parents, American Baby*, and *Reader's Digest*. Some articles have been translated into Spanish and Russian. A graduate of the Georgetown University School of Languages and Linguistics, she is a member of Phi Beta Kappa and the American Society of Journalists and Authors.

Ms. Eberlein lives in Connecticut with her husband and three children.

child

The magazine for today's parents

New solutions, fresh ideas, expert advice, good old common sense and the experiences of people like you who are raising kids in the real world. Read it first in child.

YES!

Send me a free issue of child.

If I like it I'll receive a one year subscription (10 issues in all, including my free issue) for just $8.97 — a savings of over 69% off newsstand. If I choose not to subscribe, I simply return the bill marked "cancel." The free issue is mine to keep.

To order call 1-800-777-0222 extension 1122
Rate good in U.S. only

....

Look for all the helpful books in the child magazine series

SLEEP
TANTRUMS
GOODBYES

Available from Pocket Books

POCKET
BOOKS

1220

go to bed at 8:30 so you'll feel rested for school
in the morning.